Taming the Conflict Dragon

TAMING THE CONFLICT DRAGON

Mastering Obstacles to Collaboration in the Workplace & in Life

by Alexander Hiam

Including **Wizard's Workshop** *Activities and Tools*

Produced in association with **Insights for Training & Development**
Published by **Facts On Demand Press**

Hiam, Alexander.
  Taming the conflict dragon : mastering obstacles to collaboration in the workplace & in life / by Alexander Hiam.
    p. cm.
    Includes index.
    ISBN: 1-889150-35-5

    1. Conflict management.   I. Title.

HD42.H53 2003   658.4'053
                                 QBI03-200622

Printed in USA
Published by Facts on Demand Press
www.brbpub.com
1-800-929-3811

Cover and text design: Frederick Schneider/Grafis

Preface

We have very high expectations for ourselves in the context of our work. When at work, we hope and need to get along well, to avoid anger and fighting. And we strive to achieve tough challenges through teamwork with other people, people who are often very different from ourselves.

The modern workplace is a unique invention in the history of human progress, and it demands the most and the best of its people. This is a very healthy thing. To "be all we can be" we don't necessarily need to join the U.S. Army (which used that inspiring jingle for many years). We can really sign up for any workplace where people strive together toward a worthwhile, common goal. We have the opportunity to achieve a high degree of collaboration with others, provided we learn to handle conflict especially well.

To make the best of our opportunities for greatness requires us to behave and perform at a very high level indeed, and perhaps there are few workplaces where this potential is fully achieved today. New commitments and new skills may be required, and this book and workshop are designed to offer a handful of the most important of these skills.

For in the modern workplace, people of all sorts must get along and move their work ahead in intensive collaboration with each other. What a fascinating "laboratory" in which to improve our repertoire of human skills! And what wonderful benefits accrue when we hone these skills in the context of our work, and then discover that they have at least as great a value in our families and communities as well.

Contents

ARE WE HOOKED ON CONFLICT?

Did you know that:

- 2 million violent incidents are reported each year in U.S workplaces.

- Forty-one percent of U.S. employees believe their employers do not trust them, and 62 percent do not trust their company to keep its promises.

- 1½ million workplace "simple assaults" —verbal threats and arguments— make it into police reports each year. [1]
(But how many more go unreported?)

- More than half of U.S marriages end in divorce.

- There are more than 100 million U.S. court filings each year.

- One out of every 200 Americans is shot each year. [2]

- In workplace surveys, a third to a half of employees say they are harassed, bullied, or treated rudely in their workplaces. This is one of the most common 'hidden' reasons for good employees to quit their jobs.

Introduction to the Second Edition

A recent ad in *The Wall Street Journal* for an executive course on "bargaining for advantage" at a top-ranked U.S. business school promised to teach us how to "stop leaving money on the table," "get more out of your sales force," and "regain pricing power." These power-phrases epitomize the most common management perspective on handling conflicts, disagreements, and negotiations: That by force of technique and personality, we ought to be able to exert sufficient power to overwhelm the opposition and impose our way upon them.

In the story, how-to book, and workshop materials you are holding, you will find that this tough executive approach to conflicts is rarely if ever effective. It may give the temporary illusion of victory, but it alienates those with whom you must live and work, and it also has a nasty habit of escalating the conflict until both sides are at it tooth and claw.

Which brings us around to dragons. Because in any conflict, there are the people involved. And then there is the conflict itself, which if given too much nourishment can come to life and rear up, breathing smoke and fire—to become the driving force and focus, taking control over the proceedings and leading to escalation and destruction, instead of to constructive solutions.

Several years ago, I developed a short workshop and booklet called *The Wizard's Guide to Taming the Conflict Dragon*. It shared some of the wisdom of many "wizards" I have known or whose insights I have extracted from studies of effective conflict-handling, negotiation and peace-making in the extensive literature on these subjects. The best negotiators, communicators, mediators, and team-builders take a different approach from the tooth-and-claw stereotype of the tough executive.

In fact, those who produce the best results generally do leave a little something on the table. And they do not appear to be fighting or arguing. Far from it. They maintain an emotionally comfortable context and they use a rich vocabulary of communications to reach out

1

and understand the other side's issues, as well as to share their own concerns.

Here is one fascinating fact. The best negotiators (with the most successful track records) ask far more questions than the average negotiator or executive does. Instead of declaring what they want or what "the facts" are, they ask questions.

Do we tend to ask or to tell when we are in disagreements, arguments, or negotiations? Hmm. Good question! But to answer it might take some effort because, in truth, it is hard to recall exactly how we behave under the pressure of conflict. Becoming better students of our own behavior is an essential step on the path to mastering conflict and becoming a "conflict wizard," as this mastery is represented in the book.

The true conflict wizard sees any clashing of interests with another as an opportunity, not a problem. But the wizard understands that, if not handled wisely, this opportunity can be lost and the conflict will produce a bitter harvest of problems instead.

Conflicts have great power of their own, and that this power must be respected. All one has to do is read the morning's paper to see the social and personal costs of conflicts whose power is allowed to spin out of control.

In the pages that follow, this bottled-up potential for anger and injury is symbolized by dragons. They are powerful beasts. No square-jawed executive is going to stare one down once it has been released and allowed to gain control of a conflict through careless or uninformed actions on the part of the participants.

There is truly a certain magic to the skills of the best negotiators, mediators and peace-makers. They can turn seemingly impossible situations around, bring people back together, and create new solutions to old problems. They not only tame those dragons but also help people move ahead and achieve their important objectives, even if those objectives may seem to bump head-on into the interests of other people or institutions at first.

The Conflict Dragon has come to represent the dangers as well as the opportunities of conflicts at quite a few workplaces and also at many schools, churches, and other organizations. At the U. S. Department of Agriculture, someone had the bright idea of making up actual dragons out of that squishable foam they make "stress balls" from, and circulating them with the phone number of the department's excellent Conflict Prevention and Resolution centers along with the message "Tame the Conflict Dragon" imprinted on the underbelly. I have one of these amusing stress-dragons beside me now as I write. I think I'll give it a quick squeeze to make sure I am relaxed enough to be prepared for the day's excitements and challenges, whatever they may prove to be!

Whatever your and my day's challenges do prove to be, one thing we can predict with certainty is that they will include more than a few conflicts of one sort or another. By being a highly social species, living and working in intricately interconnected groupings, we are always bumping into other parties' interests as we pursue our own.

Sometimes we have the wisdom (or magic) to align these conflicting interests and pull together with others for a while. Then our lives and our works move forward, and indeed, society itself prospers and grows. Other times, these conflicts turn into dragons and release their destructive power, hurting those involved. The damage may be limited to one individual's stress, or it may expand to effect the performances of a work group or company, the fate of a family, or, in extreme cases (yet the headlines tell us extreme cases are too common), the fate of a nation and its people. Clearly, achieving a high degree of mastery over our conflict dragons is an essential step in our advancement as a people and our success as a global economy. And, of course, it is of great benefit to us individually as we wend our individual ways along our crisscrossed career and personal paths.

My firm develops training materials and workshops that are used in thousands of workplaces, and so my focus in writing this book is mostly on conflicts in our professional lives. Yet the same skills and techniques apply elsewhere, so please feel free to bring them home or into other contexts as well. If your church group or synagogue is in a dispute, you'll find that the same principles apply as those needed to resolve a conflict with a co-worker, employee, boss, or customer. And mediators and therapists who work with families report that many of the same principles hold in those more personal and painful conflicts as well.

Because my own work is focused on adult education in the workplace, our first edition of *Taming the Conflict Dragon* was a little booklet that was not offered through bookstores. You could only get it if your employer purchased it in bulk from our warehouse. (The sole exception was the Jeffery Amherst Bookstore in Amherst Mass., which carried the booklet in a stack by the register for years and, by selling so many hundreds of them, finally managed to convince me that it could be a best-seller and ought to be reissued in this new form. Thanks to them for their vision and persistence, and I'm sorry I was such a slow learner!)

To remedy this problem and try to respond to the many requests we have had for the booklet, we are now issuing this paperback version of it in partnership with Facts on Demand Press, to be made available in bookstores as well as in workshops and courses.

And while we were at it, we decided to offer you an improved new edition, in which we added additional examples and stories in the main text of the booklet, and also a selection of some of the most powerful and popular of our workshop activities and tools. You really hold two different products in your hand. The first is a new edition of the original Conflict Dragon book, with its story and how-to tips (plus new case stories throughout). The second is a set of workshop materials that you can use on your own as a reader, or that teachers and workshop leaders can use for their assignments and group activities.

In other words, here is a new version of *Taming the Conflict Dragon* that we think will meet everyone's needs. By moving into bookstores and collaborating with a publisher, we can print a longer book that includes workshop materials and extra case-histories, and because of economies of scale we don't need to make the product expensive to the reader. In fact, some of the workshop materials in the back are similar to those a company or business school might purchase at prices far beyond the cost of this book.

The point is, while it took us a few years to figure it out, there was a better way to design, produce and distribute the product that would meet more people's needs, far better than before. Such is often the case whenever you take a clear, hard look at anything in business or in life. The world is full of opportunities to find a better way or break through an old barrier—or tame a conflict dragon.

But now let's get on to your pursuit of mastery over the challenges, barriers, obstacles and conflicts in your life. All you must do is turn the page to begin this journey.

Oh, and best of luck, wherever your path may lead. I'm honored to have this opportunity to travel with you for a brief while, and I hope to repay your interest with insights you can use throughout a long, generous and prosperous life.

Note Regarding the Endnotes: Yes, there are scholarly citations to sources in this book, along with additional comments of a more technical nature than in the text. No, I don't expect you to read them, not unless you are making a serious study of the topic. But it was important to me as an author to read extensively in the scholarly literature on the subject before writing, and it is with a sense of pride in the excellent work of many others that I anchor some of the more important learning points in this literature.

Acknowledgment:

Thanks to Stephanie Sousbies for the many contributions to this book and the multi-year project it represents.

Prologue

A Wizard Adventure

You've been hiking all day, struggling to cross a mountain range on a little-used pass. Night falls, it begins to storm, and your cloak and hood are soon dripping wet. (By the way, you are an apprentice Wizard, hence the funny outfit.)

Exhausted, you mutter a spell to waterproof your clothes, but find you are too tired even to summon enough magic for that simple trick. You realize you had better find shelter and get some rest. Rounding a bend in the steep path, you come out on a narrow ledge. A cliff falls away to your left, and to your right a sheer rock wall rises into the gloom above. Sheets of rain stream down the rock and rush along the path, making it virtually impossible to keep your footing. Panting, you try a simple encouragement charm you learned in the first year of Wizard school: "One step at a time!" It seems to help.

Inching your way along the dangerous path, you lean against the wall for support. Suddenly the rock seems to fall away beneath your arm and you tumble into the dark opening of a cave. You lie stunned on the dry stone floor for a few moments, then rise, tap your wand to summon light to its end, and peer around you.

Miraculously, you've stumbled into a comfortable cave with smooth, worn floors and arching ceilings, where you can lie protected from the storm. You unshoulder your pack, spread your cloak on a rock to dry, and unpack a basket of food and a blanket. After a quick snack, sleep overtakes you. Peace reigns in your makeshift shelter while the storm rages outside.

But soon a strange rumbling wakes you, accompanied by a flickering orange glow and the distant smell of gunpowdery smoke. Cursing your lack of caution, you realize too late that this snug cave must be the liar of a conflict dragon.

Before you can collect your belongings and escape, the dragon bursts through the entrance. It's a big dragon, and from the ruby sparks in its eyes you gather it is not in the best of tempers.

The dragon sniffs your scent, turns toward you, and opens its huge jaws to reveal rows of yard-long fangs, lit from behind by a fiery glow. Then a wisp of smoke emerges from its nostrils, accompanied by a low, rumbling groan.

You turn to run, hoping to find shelter deeper within the cave. But as you scramble down a winding passageway you can hear the dragon snorting and scuffling behind you, still growling and moaning in a peculiarly frightening manner.

Hoping the cave has another exit, you quicken your pace, but one thing nags you as you rush ahead. There was something about this dragon that caught your eye. (Your mentor Wizard told you to examine conflict dragons with great care.)

Oh yes—now you remember. Its teeth were tangled in what looked like a thick piece of rope, wound around and caught between several of its fangs. Odd, but perhaps it had been eating tethered goats from the village in the valley below and one of the tethers had gotten stuck in its mouth. Oh well, just what you need, you think—a dragon with a toothache! They are touchy enough when they're comfortable, and you suspect an uncomfortable dragon will be even harder to deal with.

Rounding a bend, you emerge in a large chamber piled high with glittering gold and silver trinkets. You've run straight to the dragon's nest. Now you're in for some serious trouble.

Scrambling over the pile, your eye is caught by a long, glittering silver sword. Grasping it, you cower behind the treasure pile and wait for the dragon's attack. Too bad you didn't have time to grab your wand, you think. A concealment spell could be handy about now. But without access to magic, you realize you'll just have to face the dragon and take your chances.

Here it comes—not rushing as you'd feared, but stalking slowly like a cat on the trail of a mouse. Silently, step by cautious step, it climbs atop its treasure nest and peers into the gloom in search for you. You squeeze between two boulders, the sword held up to protect your front, hoping you can stay out of sight. But soon one of the dragon's eyes has spotted you and it moves smoothly in your direction.

The head now looms above you, the gnarled jaws open, and you find yourself staring at its glimmering fangs, barbed tongue, and glowing throat. "All the better to eat you with" you think wildly, your mind spinning with fright.

But this is a slow-moving dragon. It seems to be toying with you, trapping you against the rock with its hot jaws while it eyes you as if wondering what you'll taste like. What if you simply thrust upward with the sword as hard as you can? You might be able to bury it in the soft pallet of the dragon's mouth—one of the few ways to kill a beast of this size.

But why would it expose this vulnerable spot to you? Was it a trick? Whatever its motives, you recognize you must act at once. If you hope to save yourself, the next move is up to you.

What will you do?

The Book

1. Dancing with the Conflict Dragon

Misunderstanding, misspeaking, blaming, disagreeing.

Disputes. Debates.

Arguments, competition, rivalry, discord, strife.

Problems, jealousy, resentment, regret.

Fear, tears, fights.

Distance. Dislike. Cruelty, put-downs, insults.

Frustrations, disappointments, complaints.

Distrust.

Avoiding, conceding, internalizing, forgetting.

Demanding, reminding, requesting, restating.

Apologizing. Suggesting. Offering.

Helping. Proposing, solving, resolving.

Returning. Revisiting. Reviving.

Conflict

2. Finding the Dragons in Your Life

Whenever one person's wishes, desires or activities bump into another's, you have a conflict of interests.

∽

What if I challenged you with three options?
They are *(I knew you'd ask)*,

1. You can live a life completely free of conflict, avoiding all disagreements and contests with others.

2. You can become so powerful that you overwhelm any objections to what you want to do with a wave of your hand, and are able to do exactly as you wish.

3. You can become so skilled at handling conflicts that you neither have to avoid them, nor win them. Instead, you can treat them as opportunities to overcome barriers to your own and other people's progress.

*O*kay, it is a bit of a stacked question, I admit. If it were a multiple choice exam, you might guess "3" even if you hadn't had a chance to study. Because neither "1" nor "2" are realistic. Oh sure, they are, superficially, quite appealing. But neither is possible, really, or if it were, it would be too much for anyone to bear for long.

To truly avoid conflicts, you would have to avoid people. Your wish could be granted only by becoming a hermit and living in isolation. That doesn't sound like fun.

To get your way in every conflict or disagreement is also superficially appealing, but ultimately, just as much a dead end. Only someone with supreme power could live this way. You'd have to be a monarch of epic proportions, with no one but "yes men" around you and everyone terrified of your next whim. It might be fun at first, but before long it would seem terribly lonely indeed.

So option "3" is much the most appealing, since we cannot truly escape from conflict, nor can we really benefit from 'winning' all conflicts. Life in human society is a collaborative venture, and, the more fully it is lived, the more often it involves conflict in some of its many forms.

There is, actually, a fourth option, and we ought to consider it because it is the one most of us choose. It is to act as if conflict is not important and does not need any special care or skills.

In this option, we go on in much the same way humans have for centuries, muddling through our disagreements and problems, sometimes poorly and sometimes well. But in the end, this "ignore it and it will go away" approach to the conflict challenge is also a losing proposition. For it means we never achieve our full potential, and often do not even see the opportunities that we leave lying on the table.

Facing the Fact of Conflict

Conflict reaches into all our daily lives, although rarely in headline-grabbing forms. Each of us has conflicts of interest with those we share our work and our lives with. In fact, most people have many minor conflicts every day—which means that even a small improvement in the quality of conflict resolutions can accumulate to make a big difference in our lives.

Yet we are accustomed to a certain amount of conflict and we do not pay much attention to routine disagreements. We rarely stop to examine our own conflict-handling behavior.

When workshop participants are asked to recall and describe recent conflicts, they usually come up with many more than they expected they would. You can try this experiment too. Just write a list of all the recent occasions in which you felt that you wanted to do something that others wanted to keep you from doing, or vice versa. (Or sometimes the conflict is over how we do the thing we want to do. Or who gets to do or have something first. Whenever there is disagreement or the potential for it, that's a conflict.)

Use the Conflict Awareness Worksheet to help you recall and describe each conflict you experienced over the past week. Or if you get inspired, just start listing conflicts on a blank sheet of paper. The worksheet's structure is only here to make it easier to get started.

CONFLICT AWARENESS WORKSHEET

1. I wanted to:

But someone else wanted to:

2. I wanted to:

But some organization or regulation stood in my way:

3. Other(s) wanted to:

But I...

4. Other(s) wanted me to:

But I...

While some of the conflicts this activity brings to the surface are relatively minor, others may be of great importance. A dispute with our boss or spouse or an unexpected experience of customer anger or someone's "road rage" can easily get under our skin, reminding us unexpectedly of how powerful and dangerous the conflict dragon can be. [3]

But whether routine and easily ignored or traumatic and hard to forget, our daily conflicts follow familiar patterns that reflect ingrained habits. As a result, we tend to repeat the same patterns in conflicts, over and over. And these patterns rarely produce optimal resolutions, for us or for the others involved.

Meet Mattie and Her Conflict Dragons

Take the example of Mattie, a teacher and the mother of two girls in their early teens. She recently filled in a conflict worksheet and thought about how she responded to the conflicts in her life. Here are some of the conflicts she listed:

> Her older daughter wants to be able to drive the car and go out at night, but Mattie doesn't feel comfortable about her driving. Besides, she thinks her daughter is seeing a much older boy that Mattie doesn't trust.

> The principal at her school wants her to teach a different grade and switch to a larger classroom next year, but Mattie is comfortable with her current assignment and does not want to have to make the change.

> Mattie's ex-husband said he would take the daughters on the weekend, so Mattie made plans to travel with a friend, but now her ex says he is busy and can't take them.

> Her teacher's aid has been suffering from allergies and asked Mattie if he could miss a few days, and not have to do the grading this coming weekend. Mattie is suspicious, however, that the aid has travel plans of his own and isn't really sick.

Students asked Mattie to be the faculty sponsor for a new photography club and she said she'd be delighted to. Then one of her colleagues got mad at her because he said she had "taken the club from him" and that "it had been his idea for the students to start it in the first place." When she asked the students if she should step aside and let him be their sponsor, they said they couldn't stand working with him because he was too controlling and they wanted her instead.

She is in a dispute with the local phone company because she found on her last bill that they were billing her for long distance calls for some other company she'd never heard of. But they say that according to some new regulation they just do the billing for long-distance carriers and it is up to her to straighten things out with them. Mattie can't reach the mysterious new company and feels that her local carrier should take responsibility.

Actually, Mattie's list could have gone on indefinitely: The woman in the grocery store parking lot who stole her space, the rude clerk at the post office, the newspaper boy who always throws the newspaper in the road instead of on her porch...she realizes that simply as a result of living and working with other people, she is often in petty conflicts with them, and sometimes in more serious ones as well. (She doesn't like to talk about her recent divorce or the many complications she runs into in trying to deal with her ex about whether he'll help with the family bills and see the children regularly. However, these are certainly serious conflicts for Mattie and her children.)

When Mattie asked herself what approach she took to her conflicts, she was not sure at first. She knew right off the bat what her ex-husband's approach was. He always seems eager to get in an argument and acts determined to win it, even if only by virtue of being the loudest.

In fact, her Principal is often competitive about conflicts too, in his own way. He never shouts, but he does tend to press his views strongly and doesn't like to give in to the teachers, or to share too much information with them.

But to Mattie, conflicts always feel uncomfortable and she prefers to try to get along with people rather than to argue with them. Mattie realizes that her preference is to avoid conflicts entirely, or if she can't avoid them, to give in. She senses that these habits often get in the way of handling her conflicts well.

For instance, she ducked the issue of how to handle her daughter's use of the car and almost told her to stop going out with that unsavory older student, but then lost her nerve and postponed the conversation. As for the other teacher who wanted to sponsor the photo club, Mattie realizes she's been avoiding him so as not to have to give him the bad news.

Mattie is becoming aware of her own particular conflict pattern, and realizes that sometimes it might be making the conflicts worse than they need to be. She, like all of us, has a pattern or style of handling conflicts, and by becoming more aware of it, she is better able to choose her response—instead of repeating the same old pattern.

What's Your Conflict Style?

Why do we repeat our same conflict patterns over and over? For lack of self-management of our own conflict behavior—an oversight the Wizard can help us solve—and also because the emotional pressure and stress of conflict situations causes us to default to ingrained responses. *(4)* We tend to have a personal conflict style that emerges when we are under pressure, whether it is the best approach to the conflict or not.

In workshops and trainings, people often fill in a survey that tells them what their habitual conflict-handling style is. (You can do this in the Wizard workshop in the back of this book.) Which of these five styles best describes you? *(5)*

Some people *avoid* conflicts, doing anything to put distance between themselves and those they are in conflict with. (Mattie's primary style is to avoid.)

Some cave in and *accommodate* or concede too quickly, preferring to let others win rather than assert themselves. (Mattie's secondary style is to accommodate, if avoiding won't work.)

Still others *compete*, fighting hard to hold their ground or beat the other person, regardless of whether fighting makes the most sense in the circumstances. Some of these competitors are aggressive about conflicts, but others are playful, haggling and bargaining whenever they have the opportunity and enjoying opportunities to use their negotiating skills.

Then there are those who prefer to *compromise*, wanting simply to split the difference and get on with it. They prefer expediency and ease of resolution.

Finally, there are those whose natural instinct is to come around to the same side of the table as the other party in the conflict and share their concerns and ideas. They like to *collaborate* in resolving the conflict. They want to make things right and will dig into the problem until they've found the most acceptable solution for all.

Mattie's conflicts include some that need firm, even competitive, handling. She probably needs to give her teenage daughter some clear rules about the car and her dating behaviors, and not to avoid this parental duty or allow herself to be talked out of it. Perhaps she needs to take a firm line with her ex-husband too. He may simply be in the habit of 'walking over her' in conflicts if she has always allowed him to in the past. Anyway, if she doesn't tell him what she wants—in this case to be able to go on her weekend trip—there is zero chance of her being able to. So avoiding will only lead to a "loss" for Mattie, while being a bit more assertive might allow things to work out better for her and the children. (Incidentally, Mattie and her "ex" may not get along in part, maybe even in large part, because of their differing conflict-handling styles. Sometimes couples save their marriages by learning to handle their conflicts more effectively.)

Mattie's relationship with her principal probably needs to be pursued in a collaborative style. If he takes an interest in her concerns (why she doesn't want to move rooms or teach a different grade), they may be able to work something out. For instance, he does not know that Mattie finds most of the rooms in the school-building too cold for her in the winter. She likes her room because she finds it cozy and warm. She would be more willing to move if she was sure the new room would be warm too.

Unless this underlying concern is discussed, the principle is not going to be sensitive to it and Mattie will not be comfortable in whatever classroom she is assigned. But, it may take some work for Mattie to get to the point where the Principal is interested in her side of the conflict; there will be more on how she overcomes this challenge in later chapters.

Similarly, the principle probably does not realize that Mattie is planning to take a course herself over the coming summer, so that this summer would be a difficult time for her to have to prepare to teach a new grade level that she has not taught before. But if she could teach one of the grades she has past experience teaching, her prep time would be less and she would be more willing to change.

In fact, Mattie would be perfectly happy to teach a new grade in a new classroom, if she and the principal could work out the details in a way that met both their needs. Like many workplace conflicts, Mattie's conflict with her boss is best resolved through collaboration. [6]

Collaboration is Great, But...

Natural collaborators want to find a way to avoid the either-or constraints of the conflict. They believe that we should reach out to each other and rise above the constraints. That's a powerful thing to do, but it is not always easy.

It takes trust-building communication skills to collaborate, and it also takes insight into the underlying interests at stake. [7] In other words, it takes advanced wizard skills to make collaboration really work. Collaboration is like magic: It's easy if you know how, but nearly impossible until you acquire the necessary techniques.

For example, take the case of Mattie's friend Jane, who Mattie is planning to go on a weekend trip with. When Mattie told her that she might not be able to go because her assistant teacher was "out sick" and her ex said he didn't want to take the girls that weekend, Jane's response to Mattie was, "OK, let's work this out. Why don't you find out what's really going on with your assistant, and also see what your husband's plans are. There must be some way three reasonable adults can find to each do what they want without getting in the way of the others. There are 52 weekends in the year, after all!"

Collaborators want us to trust and help each other. And they are right. Collaboration is the best way to achieve optimal solutions in which everyone gets as much as possible.

Yet collaborators are sometimes disappointed. Too often, others refuse to cooperate with them and they end up being taken advantage of. Or even when everyone tries to collaborate, they may fail to find a solution that makes everyone happy. So they end up back where they started, arguing over the same old things all over again.

When Mattie tried to follow her friend Jane's advice, it worked well with her assistant teacher, but not with her ex. The teacher admitted he had a new girlfriend in a distant city, and wanted to travel to spend a long weekend with her. Mattie said she didn't mind, but wanted to know in advance instead of having her assistant sneak off unexpectedly. She suggested that her assistant could take a Friday and Monday off once a month and Mattie would be happy to cover the work for him—providing she had a few weeks' advance notice.

This seemed appealing to the assistant teacher since it gave him more opportunities to travel. It also appealed to Mattie, since it gave her more control over her own schedule: A classic "win-win" solution.

And the two of them agreed to postpone the assistant's next trip for a week since Mattie had hotel reservations she and her friend could not cancel for the coming weekend. With the good news that the assistant would be able to visit his girlfriend more often, the girlfriend agreed to come to see him this weekend, so everyone ended up happy after Mattie and her assistant talked it out.

But things did not go as smoothly with Mattie's ex-husband. When she tried to explain her problem, he snapped back at her, "Why is it always about you? What if I have travel plans too?"

Mattie knew he didn't have anything planned since he'd been scheduled to take the girls that weekend. She suspected he was just trying to upset her own plans. She also was stung by the accusation that she was being selfish, since after all it was she who was raising the children and, for the most part, paying their expenses. Anyway, the conversation degenerated from there. She couldn't even remember what they'd said by the time she hung up. She did remember becoming so upset that she hung up the phone in the middle of the conversation.

Her friend Jane just looked at her, shook her head, and said, "You were supposed to find out what his plans are so we can try to work around them. Instead you ended up arguing with him again and then hanging up on him!"

"I know, I know," Mattie sighed. "But he said it 'was all about me' and then I kind of lost my head and forgot what the plan was. I always get upset when he says that."

Wizards Know What Makes Them Mad

One of the best tricks Wizards have for taming conflicts is their ability to avoid getting upset or mad. When you lose your temper, you lose control of the dragon and allow it to escalate the conflict rapidly.

So all you have to do is get rid of your temper and you can control conflicts much more easily, right? Unfortunately not. Nobody can rid themselves of their temper. Anger (like many other emotions) is a natural, physiological response. All human beings have tempers. Even Wizards have tempers. But Wizards don't lose their tempers often because they know their tempers better than most of us do.

Do you know what makes you mad? Go ahead, take a moment to think about it. Then write down a list of some of the things that are most likely to make you lose your temper. (I hope it doesn't make you mad when someone asks you what makes you mad...)

What makes me the maddest?

1. Not owning behavior
2. Not apologizing
3. Attacking Character
4. Yelling
5. Interrupting

Know them. Recognize them.
Be prepared to resist their influence.

These are your conflict dragons!

What did you come up with? Stop and look at your list carefully. Think about whether you make a special effort to be on your guard when one of those things occurs. If you prepare yourself in advance, then these things are less likely to take control over your emotions. Wizards know their own conflict dragons and are prepared to meet them anywhere.

In general, the things that make people the most mad fall into these broad categories:

> *Insults*
> *Attacks to self-esteem*
> *Injustice—unfair treatment*

Your personal conflict dragons are probably examples of one or more of these common forms. [8] Also,

> *Inability to control bad events*

is another common conflict dragon. To many people, this may feel like a form of injustice. ("It's just not fair that I can't get through to the airline when I need to change my ticket" for example.)

If a feeling of lack of control over negatives makes you mad, recognize it next time before it can take control of your mood. The person who fails to control this conflict dragon always loses their temper when driving in a traffic jam—forgetting to remind themselves that *most* of the time they are able to control their own speed and direction of travel.

A feeling of lack of control often compounds the other problems when a conflict escalates. This out-of-control feeling arises when the other party(s) in the conflict begin to get upset and flex their muscles. They become hard to control when they are upset, which in turn upsets us more, which... You get the idea. And so the conflict dance spirals ever higher.

Transforming Conflict into Opportunity

Few people actually feel in charge of their conflicts. Most feel (quite rightly) that they are frustrated or thwarted by conflicts. The conflict dragon is a wild and potentially dangerous creature, one that few but true wizards are comfortable in the presence of or able to control with ease.

Yet conflicts need not be feared and avoided. Wizards who practice the art of dragon taming learn that there is truly something magical about the potential to produce good. For example, take the case of Hamifa Cherifi, who is a full time "conflict wizard" in the Education Ministry in Paris. Her specialty is helping resolve the conflicts that too often arise when the children of Muslim immigrants bring their faith and traditions to French schools.

For instance, the teachers and administrators in many communities throughout France take objection to Muslim girls wearing head scarfs. And when these children are sent home with instructions not to wear their traditional headgear to school, the families sometimes object strongly on religious or cultural grounds. Behind this objection is the reality that many of these Muslim immigrants feel they are already being discriminated against, and that this school rule is a challenge because it fits the broader pattern of discrimination against them and their children.

Sometimes the child will have been forced to sit alone in an empty classroom for weeks on end by the time Ms. Cherifi finally arrives (according to a report in *The Wall Street Journal* dated June 26 '03). And teachers have also been known to go out on strike if local authorities order them to permit a child to wear a scarf in school.

So this is no small disagreement, this is the stuff of serious conflicts, with tempers and prejudices rising high and both sides determined not to give in. There is a stronger belief in the idea that newcomers should integrate into French society by adopting the country's customs and language than we are used to now in the United States, so these conflicts are especially difficult. Yet similar conflicts arise in U.S. schools and workplaces as well.

How does Ms. Cherifi resolve these conflicts? By doing a lot of listening to both sides. And also by trying to get more and better communications going. And she is usually able to get the child accepted in a classroom, avoiding further interruptions in her education. Sometimes the family backs down, other times the school gives in.

Whether or not someone wears a headscarf is a hard thing to negotiate, because it is either off or on. Many conflicts are more multidimensional, making it easier to find a resolution that makes both sides feel like winners. Yet even in Ms. Cherifi's tough cases, it is possible to improve the situation for both sides:

- When the student is able to sit down in the classroom and learn alongside others, that is a victory for the family and a big improvement for the student—who did not enjoy being the focus of anger and disciplinary action, to say the least.

- And when even an uneasy truce is agreed to by the teachers and administrators of the school, they can get back to teaching and administrating and no longer be caught up in a draining and disruptive conflict, so they are happier too.

The good communication skills and patience of the mediator make these positive developments possible, even though the people in the conflict usually presumed that there was no way to work things out. Why do people so often think the situation is hopeless before the Wizard arrives? Because they are too caught up in it, too caught up in their dance with the conflict dragon to see any alternatives.

When resolved in a certain way, conflicts produce innovative, growth-oriented solutions. They lead to valuable breakthroughs in personal or professional life. Resolving conflict not only solves the immediate problem, it also helps all the participants gain confidence and break through their own barriers to find new and better ways to live and work.

So by mastering the conflict-handling arts, you can acquire the magical ability to turn points of friction into sources of growth and development, both for yourself and for those around you. Wizards harness the pent-up energy of conflicts to achieve breakthrough progress.

And if that's not magic, what is?

"Mine!" "No, MINE!"

A simple story is sometimes told to illustrate the hidden potential in conflicts. Once two sisters argued over an orange, each claiming they needed it more. Their mother finally imposed a compromise. She cut the orange in half. Whereupon one girl squeezed her half and drank the juice, but the other girl grated the rind of her half to use in baking a cake.

The girls were too angry with each other to talk about what they wanted the orange for, or they might have found this "obvious" solution themselves. If the girls had understood each others' needs more clearly, they could have avoided the entire argument and each gotten twice as much of what they wanted. But conflicts are often like that. It is hard to find the hidden "win-win" potential in them.

And in messy, real-world conflicts, sometimes you need to work hard to explore all the complex needs and interests—*as in the case of the tardy employee...*

3. The Case of the Tardy Employee

The manager of an administrative office at a phone company was ready to fire one of his employees because she kept coming to work late. He'd spoken to her, filed reports, done everything he could think of to change her behavior. She'd promised repeatedly she'd work on it, only to slip back into showing up late again.

In this conflict, the two parties are arguing over time, not oranges, but the root of the problem is basically the same:

Not enough to go around!

When that's the case, people typically get into a tug of war over what there is, instead of trying to find ways to create more. Only when you look beneath the surface of the conflict can you see opportunities to get more for both.

Obviously you cannot expand time itself (any more than you can make one orange into two oranges). But on some level, there is always something that can be expanded to satisfy both parties' needs more fully. So let's explore this conflict a little more deeply.

The employee's name is Darleen. She is a single mom who has to get her kids off to daycare before she goes to work — something she has not told her manager out of fear that he will hold it against her. Daycare starts at 7:30 and work starts at 8:00 am. Unfortunately, it often takes 40 minutes or more to get from day-care to work. Sometimes she drops the children off early, but that makes the director of the day-care center mad because the teachers don't arrive until opening time. (When the director has to watch the early arrivals, it keeps her from her daily set-up activities. Everyone has their own interests, don't they?)

Back at the office, the manager, whose name is Robert, likes everyone to get in early. Customer calls begin to ring through to the office by 8:30, and he likes to have a half hour in advance to run periodic staff meetings or to give people time to get on top of any leftover paperwork from the day before. To Robert, on-time arrival is an important issue and he does not want one tardy employee to set a bad example that will lead others to think they can be late too.

By the way, you ought to know that Robert was promoted to management just six months ago, and still lacks confidence in his ability to keep everything under control. This might make him more touchy about the occasional late arrival than a more secure manager would be. Everyone has their own perspective, and sometimes that means something can be a bother or a problem for one person, even though it might no seem very important to others.

Rejecting the Obvious Solutions

In this conflict, there is no way to divide the time so as to meet all participants' needs. The employee cannot drop the kids on time at day care and still be on time for work. So the participants in this conflict are heading toward a brick wall. Unless they find a way to redefine their conflict, a win-lose resolution is inevitable.

Win-lose is when one person's needs are met at the expense of the other's. If Robert gives in and lets Darleen continue to be late, he will lose. If he fires her for being late, then she will lose. But there is more to the win-lose equation than that.

In Win-Lose Solutions, *Everybody* Loses Something

In a less obvious way, both of them will lose from either of the obvious win-lose outcomes. Robert wins the conflict, to be sure, if he fires Darleen. But he'll be short one tardy but otherwise good employee and will need to go through the trouble and expense of hiring and training someone new. So there are large hidden costs to him in that win-lose scenario.

There are also hidden costs for Darleen if she wins at the expense of Robert. Even if Robert concedes and grudgingly lets her get away with being tardy for a little longer, Darleen will continue to wrestle with the stress of this problem. That, combined with the likelihood of an increasingly frosty relationship with her boss, will guarantee a stressful life and make Darleen feel insecure about her job. And she certainly is not going to get a good performance review from Robert or have a chance to advance or get a raise if she continues to be in violation of her employer's policies.

So to avoid significant costs from this conflict, the participants have to do some creative problem solving. They have to come up with a new approach, which means they will have to share information about their needs and constraints, then join forces to help each other. And they may need to reach out and seek outside help too.

Unfortunately, most conflicts are never resolved in an optimal manner. Usually, the participants fail to explore each other's (or their own) positions fully. And they rarely sit down and join forces to try to find new ways to solve each other's problems. But if they did, even as tough a problem as this one might be solvable.

Listing the Underlying Interests

Fortuitously in the case of the tardy employee, the participants happened to be in a workshop on conflict management, and they applied the Wizard's methods to their own problem. The Wizard told them a little-known rule of conflict resolution, which is that:

Conflicts are never about what you think they are.

So they stopped and asked themselves, and each other, what this conflict was really about.

And in the resulting discussion, Darleen and Robert realized that, contrary to what they had both believed, they were not arguing over time at all. Instead, their real interests were:

To make sure the children don't lose their places at a good daycare,

To make sure the employee doesn't miss staff meetings or fall behind on her paperwork, and

To avoid setting a precedent in the office that might lead other employees to think they can get away with arriving late.

These are the key interests at stake in this conflict. They were hidden beneath the dispute over whether Darleen could get away with arriving fifteen minutes late.

Notice that Darleen and Robert did not write two opposing lists, as would be natural to do in a conflict. They just wrote one list. The list has each of their most important interests on it. If the two of them can find a mutually agreeable way to satisfy each of the concerns on this list, then everyone can walk away from the conflict happy.

Conflict Wizards believe that you cannot seek true solutions until everyone is looking at the same list. Otherwise, each party to the conflict is working on solving a different problem, which makes it hard to solve any problem well.

Once Darleen and Robert put their shared list of underlying interests on the table, they were no longer locking horns on the one-dimensional and unsolvable issue of arrival time. And they were no longer each pursuing different concerns and solutions without the help of the other. Now they could both see the full problem, not just the side of it visible from their own position.

There is a useful principle here that Conflict Wizards always employee in dragon-taming:

**As soon as you clarify the underlying interests,
you can begin exploring the conflict in new ways.**

Conflict dragons like to hide the true nature of conflicts behind their smoke and fire. One of the Wizard's best "magic tricks" is to sit down with the other person in a conflict and write an accurate list of each other's underlying needs or interests, just as Robert and Darleen did in the case of the tardy employee. When you make the underlying interests and concerns visible, new possibilities beyond the original "my version your version" struggle begin to appear. [9]

Achieving Insight

In the case of the tardy employee, once Robert understood Darleen's concerns about day-care, then he was able to begin helping her solve her problem. It was no longer a case of a disobedient employee. It was now a case of a good employee who had a difficult problem that got in the way of her arriving on time. How to solve that problem?

Similarly, once Darleen understood Robert's concerns about her not missing staff meetings and about not setting a bad precedent that would lead to others arriving late too, then she was able to focus on how to solve Robert's problem. She no longer thought her boss was "a jerly" she understood that Robert had some legitimate concerns too.

They had seen through the smoke. They had achieved insight into the true nature of the conflict. They were ready to collaborate to tame this conflict dragon!

What did they do? It took some time and work, but in the end they invented a solution that was satisfactory to everyone, and that prevented the obvious alternative of Robert having to search for a new employee and Darleen having to search for a new job:

- Darleen found one of the day-care teachers was willing to come in early two days a week for a small fee, which allowed Darleen to make it to all staff meetings on time.

- Robert agreed to give Darleen advance notice of a week or more when scheduling staff meetings so she could arrange the early day care for her children and be there on time.

- On days when there was not a staff meeting, Robert agreed to let Darleen come fifteen or twenty minutes late, so long as she stayed equally late that day to finish all her paperwork.

- Robert circulated a memo to the rest of the people at the employee's office. The memo explained the special arrangement, and also made it clear that the arrival time was still 8:00 for other employees unless they too came forward with unusual and pressing needs and were able to make a special arrangement with Robert.

- Also, Darleen and Robert both agreed do some research to see if they could find a day-care option Darleen approved of that was nearer to the office and easier to get to. They hoped that a better option might be found in time, but with the compromise they worked out, there was no rush to move the children until another good daycare could be found.

Happy Endings!

Job saved. Conflict dragon defeated. Everybody happy. But it was a very close call. Only expert conflict-handling skills can solve problems as tough as that one. It takes skills like using one's Wizard insight to look beneath the surface of a conflict and find out what the underlying interests really are.

And to do that—to gain insight into the true nature of a conflict so you can apply your problem-solving skills to it—we need to break down the normal barriers of communication. Instead of arguing about the conflict, we need to clear the smoke and exchange honest, accurate information about underlying interests.

What if the other person doesn't want to do that? Or what if your own emotional reaction gets in the way of your doing it? To make sure you get onto the right pathway, the Wizard recommends you automatically switch mental gears whenever you enter a conflict. As soon as it is clear you are in a conflict situation, experienced conflict wizards recommend you switch to a style of communication called reflective listening.

4. Reflective Listening

*"Empathy requires enough calm receptivity so that the subtle sig-
nals of feeling from another person can be received and mimicked
by one's emotional brain."*
　　　　—Daniel Goleman, *Emotional Intelligence,* 1995, p. 104
∿

Q uiet your mind until it is as still and open as a calm pool of
water. Then let them look within the pool. What do they see?

When you give others glimpses of themselves in your mirror, you
gain insight into their interests and feelings. And they gain insight too.

People are rarely clear on what their interests are in a conflict.
Often, it is not possible at first to sit down and write that single list of
both parties' underlying needs and concerns because the other party
is not yet ready to do so. You can't work on a resolution until you help
them get clear on what they need. So reflection leads to valuable
insights into the true nature of a conflict. And it helps build trust and
openness between you, clearing the way toward resolution. [10]

There are two principle ways to build trust: by communicating in
a concerned, trusting manner, and by behaving consistently and con-
siderately. Reflection taps into both of these trust-building techniques.

The Magic of Opening and Inviting

How do you unleash the magic of reflection? By opening yourself
to the other person's concerns, and then by inviting them to express
those concerns to you.

You can open and invite nonverbally, simply by feeling open and interested in their concerns. To do so, ask yourself these simple questions:

"Why are they concerned?"

"What are their underlying interests?"

These questions focus you on their underlying motives, rather
than the surface impression made by their visible behavior.

Your efforts to understand their behavior open you up by tapping into your natural ability to empathize, or to "put yourself in their shoes." Why do that? Because in conflict, the only way to make peace is to "know your enemy." Asking yourself "Why do they behave as they do?" leads you to consider their motives, which is the essential first step toward optimal resolution.

Listening with Questions

As we've just seen, it is entirely possible to reflect on the conflict on your own. You don't really need their cooperation or participation in the beginning. However, it is often helpful to use reflective listening statements and questions—which gets them more actively involved in the reflection process.

To use words to invite them into the reflection, you might try something like these examples:

Say this to signal openness:	Then say this to invite expression:
I feel like you might be upset.	Can you tell me how you feel?
I didn't realize you disagreed.	Why don't you like this plan?
I didn't expect you to say no.	Can you tell me why?

Then, once you've signaled your openness and invited them to share their concerns with you, prepare to count to three.

Yes, three. Three rounds of conversational exchange with them, that is. Because odds are they won't pick up on your signal at first, and will reply with something that is not an open expression of their real concerns. Most likely, they will attack you on something peripheral or irrelevant to the real issue. They might come back with an irritated, "What do you care? You're the one who's causing the problem!" or something like that. So count "one" for that reply, and rephrase your open invitation statement in a calm tone of voice.

You aren't upset, because you knew they might not realize you were sincere the first time. So you can easily let their zinger whistle right past you without being effected. You won't answer it at all. You will simply issue your invitation again. (You might say something like "I understand your feeling irritated, but I really do want to know what's up here? Do you mind just going over it with me for a minute?")

Maybe they now get it and realize it is safe to open up to you and express their real feelings and concerns. But maybe they come back with a second attacking statement. If so, you still aren't upset, because you are prepared to count to three and this is just round two.

Rephrase or repeat your signal of openness now for the third time. Maybe say something like, "I can't see how to help unless I understand what's going on more clearly. What exactly is your concern?" (Notice that you use "I" not "you" to make your point. We'll talk more about the use of I phrases to avoid the 'hot button' of phrases about the other person in a later chapter.)

Most people will, at least by their third response to your opening invitation, begin to respond in kind with helpful details about their concerns. They will begin to do as you invited them: To tell you about the conflict from their perspective. After all, you did invite them "in" three times, and that's a very open and friendly way to handle someone who has a complaint or grievance. It almost always does the trick and gets them started in a real conversation with you in which some of the barriers are beginning to come down.

If they are hot-headed or really stubborn, perhaps they'll go for one more round. And then you must make a difficult choice, based on how you are feeling at the moment. Do you have the patience to tolerate a fourth angry response from them without losing your temper and saying something angry or destructive back to them? Maybe. But to be honest, I seriously doubt it. By now, almost everyone would be feeling a little irritated and heated toward this person who keeps spurning their well-meaning invitations to talk and, instead, hurls angry accusations and complaints back at them!

If you are beginning to mirror their anger by the end of the third round, be very careful what you say. You probably cannot continue to invite them into a calm conversation about their concerns. Strong emotions inevitably spread between people, and your angry "opponent" in the conflict has strong negative feelings right now that inevitably will infect you too, whether you want them to or not. That is why conflict wizards count to three. They know that no one, not even the most experienced mediators and negotiators, can be subjected to anger or insults forever without beginning to lose their own tempers. What separates the skilled conflict-wizard from the ordinary person is that the wizard realizes conflicts cannot be resolved in anger, and is therefore very careful to avoid situations and conversations that lead into anger.

So, if they are still acting angry, you could try saying something like, "I really do want to help resolve your concerns, but I need to understand exactly what your concerns are. If you are willing to talk right now, let's go for it. But I don't want us to get angry with each other, so it might be better to wait until later. Can we talk about this tomorrow afternoon?"

Now if they come back with another closed sort of answer, if they still seem too irritated to really share their true concerns in a helpful manner, you can postpone the conversation politely by making it clear you won't talk to them about it any more right now, but that you want to discuss it at a later time. In doing this, simply state what you will and won't do. Again, don't tell them what you think of them, what they are doing, or what you wish they would do. Avoid using the word "you" and it is easy to steer clear of such traps.

A simple self-descriptive statement works best, something like "I am sorry but I'm not willing to talk about it any more right now. What I am willing to do is to discuss it tomorrow afternoon." This is, of course, another type of invitation, and again, they may in anger spurn it. But even if they say, "You are a ****ing idiot and by tomorrow afternoon my lawyer is going to have you so tangled in knots you won't know which way is up," don't say anything else. Just let them know when you want to talk again.

In time, perhaps in just an hour or two, they will realize that you were being pretty reasonable and that they were making a fool of themselves, and they will remember that you said you were willing to talk again later on. Most likely, a much better-behaved and perhaps even apologetic person will approach you to see if you are still willing to talk to them tomorrow afternoon.

But this is the worst-case scenario, when the other person or people in a conflict are so unruly that they insist on dancing with conflict dragons and will not open up and accept your invitation to tell you their concerns.

Most people are pleasantly surprised, even amazed, when you show a genuine interest in their problems or concerns. They quickly realize that they have found a rare soul who is willing to listen to them complain, and who does not seem to insist on making them listen to his or her complaints. Most people will quickly begin to share their concerns, allowing you to begin to understand what the real underlying issues in the conflict are. And in many cases, they will see the wisdom in identifying the underlying issues and even in joining you as you attempt to define their concerns. And once your list of their concerns is perfected and you have helped them understand and explain what they most want or need and why the conflict concerns them— well, then, it is a natural thing for them to do the same for you and for you to begin to add your own concerns to the bottom of the list. Reflective listening first clarifies the other party's concerns, and then, by so doing, clears the air to permit you to show them what your needs or concerns are too.

And once everyone has a clear view of the real, underlying interests and concerns, the conflict may well begin to "solve itself" as possible solutions begin to become visible to all concerned.

When you make your interest in someone else's concerns clear, then they are usually willing to examine their own concerns and to help you examine them too. So this little technique can work wonders in a conflict situation.

However, it can be very difficult to open and invite when a conflict takes you by surprise. The natural defensive instinct is to close and reject instead. You can only open and invite if you believe that you gain insight and take control of the conflict by so doing. Believing you can control the conflict gives you control over your response to it.

SURPRISING BUT TRUE

Myth: We are unkind to those we dislike because they deserve it.

Fact: We dislike people because we are unkind or aggressive toward them. Aggression and discrimination create dislike. Past aggression increases our negative attitudes toward those we are aggressive to. Why? Because dislike often arises subconsciously as an emotional justification of negative treatment. Then those negative attitudes toward the victims make it more likely we'll behave negatively toward them again, creating a cycle of aggression and justification that eventually polarizes our world into clearly labeled "Good" and "Bad" people. *(11)*

---

5. Taking Emotional Control of the Conflict

The Language of Conflict:
Opponent, foe, rival, enemy, antagonist, rival, trouble-maker

The Language of Reconciliation:
Cooperator, partner, colleague, collaborator, problem-solver

What emotional responses do these words evoke in you?

~

When others oppose us, we feel like we have lost control of our ability to take care of our own interests. They—and even more the conflict itself—are suddenly seizing control. Anxiety, anger, fear and frustration feed on feelings of lost control. These negative feelings are natural responses to the wild conflict dragon that is intruding into our affairs.

We can only regain our sense of control and mastery of the situation by controlling that wild dragon. And dragons feed on emotions, so it is essential to focus on controlling the source of our feelings.

Opening and inviting are taming techniques. They give us more control over the conflict dragon by helping us achieve insight and understanding. People who use reflective listening soon learn to trust their ability to regain control of the situation.

If you say to yourself, "Oh, that must be a conflict dragon! If I am very careful and quiet, I should be able to tame it," you will be emotionally prepared to use reflective listening. But we don't always have the presence of mind to recognize a conflict dragon when we see it.

Preventing Defensive Spirals

What happens if you say to yourself something like, "That's not fair! Why is s/he getting mad at me / being mean to me / being unfair to me / blocking me / being unfriendly to me / resisting us / stalling our plans / not helping out?" These common thoughts engage associated feelings of injury and trigger natural defensive reactions.

When you use words that permit your natural defensive reactions to kick in, you will automatically respond defensively, which fuels the conflict dragon's fire by guaranteeing a defensive response from the other person in return.

Then both of you will close instead of open. Nobody will reflect. Nobody will really listen. And the conflict dragon will take advantage of the smoke to draw nearer.

Here is a fascinating fact. [12] Did you know that:

In almost every conflict, both parties believe that they are defending and the other is attacking.

~

That can't be true, of course. Yet the most obvious alternative is not true either.

We generally assume that one person must be right. So one of the people in a conflict is attacking and the other defending. But that's not true either. The definition of a conflict of interest is simply that people (or their organizations and institutions) have conflicting interests. Their interests have bumped into each other, like two trucks that want to use a narrow roadway at the same time to go opposite directions.

Let's explore the example of two trucks, traveling in opposite directions, both wanting to use a one-way road at once. Regardless of which driver might make the stronger claim to right of way, the immediate situation is simply that both cannot take up the same space at the same time, and so their desires are both thwarted by the presence of the other. (By the way, this situation was simulated in a classic set of experiments, and subjects quickly escalated into competitive efforts to keep the other truck from using the road. As a result, neither truck was able to complete its runs and do its work successfully!)

Both the drivers in this situation feel threatened by the presence of the other. Any aggressive actions either driver takes will be a response to that sense of feeling thwarted and threatened by the situation. In other words, both are initially defending their own interests, and if you ask them to describe the situation, they will say that the other truck is in their way. They see the other party as the cause and source of the problem. That is how most conflicts start. Then what one party does to defend its interests (as it sees them) feels like an attack to the other party, and vice versa. So the first defensive responses generate

stronger ones and the conflict spirals into what might look to out
siders like two parties attacking, not defending. Still, at their heart,
conflicts are about both parties' desire to defend their own interests.

Listening to Break the Cycle

Reflective listening breaks into this defensive cycle of escalating
conflict. By stopping to open, breath, invite and consider, you reveal to
yourself and others the concealed truth that you all feel you have legitimate interests to protect. Reflective listening tames the conflict dragon by making it clear you are both defending, not attacking. That is
what you both see when you look at the reflection in your open mind.

Listening to Build More Trust

The more important a conflict is to you, the less you trust the
other person. People with high stakes in a conflict develop strongly
biased views of their opponents. Their biases make it hard to believe
the opponent's statements, proposals or suggestions. And as conflict
escalates, biases and mistrust do too. [13]

This mistrust blocks open communication and prevents people
from discovering their opponents' true interests. Reflective listening
can break the escalation of mistrust by revealing the real people
behind our conflict-induced biases.

TIP

Not sure if you are fully open and receptive enough for reflective
listening? Check your hands. If your hands are fully open and
relaxed, your mind and heart are too. If your hands are clenched,
tight, cold, hot or otherwise uncomfortable, then you are not yet
ready to reflect. (And your jaw may be grinding or your face
flushed too—what are your most common physiological stress
responses?) So don't respond at all until you are physically ready
to be open. Take a few seconds (or more if necessary) to stretch,
massage or shake out your hands, and breath calmly and deeply,
before you trust yourself to reply reflectively.

---

6. Clarifying the Reflection

What you both see at first may not be very clear. Be prepared to work a little for your insight. You may need to actively reflect what the other seems to be saying in order to check that the reflection is clear. The Wizard calls this clarifying the reflection with fact-checking.

Fact-checking is when you ask them if something you think they are saying or feeling is true. It often goes something like this:

> **"It sounds to me like you are most concerned about _____. Is that right?"**

Or it might sound like this:

> **"Are you saying that you are upset about _____ because it threatens your _____?"**

As these examples show, your questions take the form of restatements of how they feel, especially how they feel about underlying needs and interests. If they agree with one of your fact-check statements, then you are both clear on that concern. Great! Now you just need to check to see if there are any other concerns. That's pretty easy too. Just say something like,

> **"Are there any other concerns?"**

Or you might feel it necessary to be more specific; something like:

> **"Okay, we're clear on that issue, and I'd like to talk about how to deal with it in a minute, but first, is it your main concern? Or are there any other issues we need to focus on?"**

When you continue to probe and explore, you will soon have a very clear picture of the other person's underlying concerns and interests. You'll know why they reacted defensively, which is half of the reason you are in conflict with them. The other half of the reason is of course your own underlying interests, but these should come clearer to you through the reflective listening process too.

When you can see their interests clearly, then you can see what part of their interests bumped into your interests. You will reveal the true nature of the conflict—which is always something different from what presented itself on the surface. So reflective listening is really just as much a selfish strategy as it is an altruistic one. By clarifying their interests, you also clarify the conflict between your interests and theirs. And that prepares you to move ahead toward an optimal resolution.

A Case in Point

Remember Mattie, the teacher who is in conflict with her principal over his telling her she has to teach a new class next year? She is upset because she likes her classroom (it is warmer than most of the classrooms), and also because she is planning to be busy over the summer and so does not look forward to having to study to prepare for teaching a new class level. Her first instinct (since she tends to avoid or accommodate in conflicts) was not to talk to the principle at all, but she knew that was not going to help her solve her problem. So her next idea was to ask for a one-on-one meeting in which she would explain her issues and ask the principal not to reassign her.

However, just as she was walking into the principal's office, she realized that she had no idea what had motivated him to want to reassign her in the first place. She knew she had been doing a great job with her 6th grade classes for the last few years. Why would he want to mess with success, as the old expression goes? Mattie decided that, before she started petitioning for her own interests, she would use active listening to find out what was on his mind. Probably he did not mean to attack her or cause her problems. Perhaps he had some concerns of his own.

At first he was somewhat hesitant to go into details, replying to her questions with guarded statements such as, "Well, Mattie, as you know I have a lot of planning to do for next year, and it's my job to wrestle with the schedules and assignments until I have everything covered adequately." This did not tell her anything—except, perhaps, that he did have some kind of problem but was not eager to share it with her.

However, Mattie figured that, if she could ask enough questions, she would eventually get to the bottom of it. After all, she and her boss were on pretty good terms and had worked together for many years now, and she did not think he would flat-out refuse to talk to her or throw her out of his office. So she kept asking in different ways, as politely as she could, and trying to gather more information about his decision. She asked about other teachers and their room and class

………………… He hedged a bit on that one but did say that there were going to be quite a few changes. She asked if they were going to be losing some of their teachers. He said, well, in fact, yes, but he could not tell her who as it was not yet formally decided.

This lead to Mattie asking if they were getting any new teachers. The principal said, yes, again it was not finalized but that he did expect to be hiring at least a couple new teachers for next fall.

Mattie, sensing she might be getting warm, asked some more questions about these new teachers. What classes or topics did they have experience teaching? Were there any subjects or levels that they were not qualified to teach? Could this be part of the principal's decision-making?

"Well, you certainly are persistent today!" the principle said, leaning back in his swivel chair and laughing. "Yes, you're right. I haven't signed the contract yet, but it looks like I may be bringing in a new teacher who has been an assistant in a 6th grade classroom in another school, but has never taught anything else. So I figure I'll need to assign him to your 6th grade class if he is going to be able to handle a classroom on his own. And since you have a lot of experience, I figured you could easily switch to another grade level if need be, so that I can work out the staffing for next year using the people I have available. All of this is confidential, by the way, Mattie. I don't want the 'rumor mill' starting. In a few weeks I'll get the contracts formalized and then I can make an announcement about it."

Mattie, being a teacher and never without pencil and paper, had been making a little tick mark on a yellow pad each time she asked her boss another question. She glanced down at it and smiled to herself. It had taken 21 questions for her to get to the bottom of the principal's actions and to begin to understand his concerns. Reflective listening was not as easy as she had expected. It certainly took some patience when dealing with a rumor-shy administrator who didn't want to share all of his information with his staff. But now she felt she did understand his underlying interest. Just to be sure, she asked one more question, designed to clarify her own understanding:

"Okay," she said, "As I understand it, and this is in confidence since it is not yet for sure, you think you'll be bringing in a new teacher who is only qualified to teach 6th grade, so you are thinking of switching me to another grade. Probably one of the grades where you expect to lose a teacher. Right?"

The principle nodded.

"And I bet you aren't in a position to tell me exactly which classes are going to lose their teachers, if you aren't sure about it yet, since that would mean breaking the confidentiality of your discussions with someone else? Although I don't know what harm there is in our knowing that someone has taken a new job at another school, I mean, we're all going to find out pretty soon anyway if it's true."

"Well," the principle said, looking cautiously around and lowering his voice, "If, just for example, there was some sort of issue with an employee, for instance, let's just say there was a chance of someone being terminated, well, that would be a serious thing and I obviously couldn't reveal anything about it during the process. I'm just giving that as an example, mind you, of how someone in my position has to maintain confidentiality about certain things that might be in an employee's file."

Now Mattie had a further insight into the principal's situation, and decided to clarify it too. She said, "So not only do you have this concern about a possible new teacher with limited qualifications and experience, but you also may have some need to maintain strict confidentiality about the future of some of our current teachers and whether they might be back next year or not. Right?"

"Yes," the principal agreed, "I am somewhat constrained by the circumstances and I have not shared all my thinking and information with the teachers in our weekly staff meetings for that reason. It's not that I want to cause you any trouble, Mattie, it's just that I have some difficult circumstances I have to deal with."

"Well, you have been very helpful and I appreciate your being willing to tell me as much as you can," Mattie said. "Can I think about this and maybe talk to you again in a day or two?"

"Sure," he said. "My door is always open. Actually, to be honest, it's not, but you can come on in if my secretary says I'm not seeing someone else or tied up on the phone or something. I'll tell him I want to see you again this week if we can fit it in. And thanks for being so understanding, Mattie. I wasn't looking forward to this meeting with you, because I expected you to be angry with me or to say you wanted to file a grievance or something."

"No problem!" Mattie said, smiling. "See you later."

What About My Concerns?

Like many of the Wizard's best tricks, reflective listening only has magical power when it is used to help someone else, rather than yourself. The Wizard is happy to grant us the power to grant other people's wishes—but not our own. This may seem disappointing at first.

When people first try to use reflective listening, they find themselves wanting to talk about their own concerns instead of the other person's. This is a natural response. In fact it is typical of almost every conflict.

When thwarted by another or faced with another's accusation or complaint, we may feel the urge to "state our case" strongly in words such as one of the following:

> **"That's not true!"**
>
> **"But you said if I _____, you'd _____."**
>
> **"I can't take that project on right now. When will I have time to do the other jobs I'm responsible for?"**
>
> **"I thought it was my turn to _____."**
>
> **"That's impossible." (Many things see impossible when we are negative about them—but it is amazing what becomes possible if our attitude changes.)**
>
> **"I always get stuck with _____."**
>
> **"Sorry, but I can't..."**
>
> **"If you _____, I may have to _____."**
>
> **"I can't see how we'd be able to help you with that."**
>
> **"No way."**
>
> **"No."**
>
> **"Absolutely not."**

Such responses are usually blurted out with only the minimum forethought and control. They can just pop into our heads or onto our tongues, perhaps surprising us as much as the other person. Where do they come from?

They come from our underlying interests asserting themselves. A little voice is crying out somewhere deep down inside us, letting us know it has just been bumped and wants us to push back to make it a little more room.

So we push back—and bump our underlying interests into their underlying interests once again. Then more complaints, more pushing, more bumps. The conflict dragons get their entertainment, but we don't get an optimal solution.

The trouble with asserting yourself quickly and strongly is that it inevitably escalates into conflict—unless the other person is a good reflective listener. And since reflective listening is a sophisticated skill, that's not very likely. You cannot count on the other person to clarify the conflict for you. Yet throwing your concerns at them is giving up your control and leaving it to them to figure out how to initiate resolution.

Exercising Leadership in Conflict

Do you want to be in charge of your own conflict or not? To take charge, to take the lead, you must explore the other party's concerns before your own.

Listen first. Listen fully. Build understanding. Let your concern with their position lay the foundations of trust and cooperation. In time it will be your turn. All in good time. Whenever you go to the trouble of surfacing the other party's concerns through reflective listening, you find that their interest in your concerns grows and they become gradually easier to collaborate with. Your good example provides conflict leadership, turning what was initially a win-or-lose conflict into an opportunity for both of you to gain.

Mattie took the lead when she used her reflective listening and fact-checking skills to find out more about her Principal's situation. In fact, as you recall, she used her first meeting with him only to ask questions and learn about his underlying interests. It was not easy to do this, even though Mattie and her boss had worked together well for some years. His concerns about avoiding rumors among the faculty, maintaining confidentiality regarding other employees, and handling next year's staffing problems combined with his natural tendency to be a "competitor" in style—meaning that he does not instinctively share information and seek help from the other party.

Mattie is, naturally, most interested in her own concerns. She does not want to have to take on a new class next year, if it means she will have to do a lot of background preparation over the summer. Nor does she want to have to teach in a drafty, chilly room, since she gets cold and depressed easily in the winter. These are her concerns. What about them? Should she now assert them strongly to her boss? She wonders how best to approach her next meeting with him.

In discussing the situation with her friend Jane on their weekend trip, Mattie explained what she had learned about the Principal's concerns. Jane's response was, "So what, Mattie? You've been there for ten years and you were teacher of the year two years ago. Shouldn't your desires have some weight too?"

Mattie thought about that. Was it now time to go back to her boss and assert her own interests? But she did not really think that was wise. What would he do? At best, he would take her concerns into consideration—adding them to his already lengthy list of problems needing to be solved. She thought that it was up to her to continue to take the lead. She explained this feeling to Jane, saying, "I don't know, Jane, I think if I push too hard now, he'll just clam up again. And I really don't have the power to make my boss do it my way, after all. I want to try to come up with some good options for him before I talk to him again."

"Options? What options can there be?" Jane said, puzzled. "I mean, either he is going to reassign you or not, and I think you'd better make it very clear to him that he'll have trouble if he tries to."

Matie was quiet for a while. Her friend had, after all, put her finger on a critical question. What other options could there be? If she couldn't come up with any more, then it was going to come down to her way or her boss's way, and she had a hunch who was going to win out in that sort of either-or situation. But why couldn't there be other approaches? If she knew nothing else about the process of assigning teachers and classrooms, she knew it was complex. And complex was good, she thought, because it meant that there were probably many ways to do it. And one of those ways, she hoped, might meet both her own and her Principal's needs.

Now that Mattie understands her boss's issues and constraints more fully, she is in a position to transform the conflict into a puzzle that she (and he) may be able to solve in new and better ways for them both. Her thinking is moving naturally to the next step in a good conflict-handling process. She is on the verge of transforming the initial conflict, rather than accepting it as it was presented.

"You see," Mattie explained to Jane, "one of the fundamental rules of conflict management is that conflicts are never about what you think they are. And I think that means it's up to me to come up with a better way to define this conflict."

"But what about your concerns?" Jane persisted. "You're not running a charity here, you're trying to keep from getting screwed by your boss!"

"I don't think he meant it as an attack on me at all," Mattie said. "He's just struggling to solve some very real staffing problems for next year. I'm going to give him the benefit of the doubt and see if by helping him, I can help myself in the bargain."

"Okay, maybe you are right," Jane said. "But still, I'd love to get a chance to go a few rounds with him. You're not assertive enough, Mattie. If it were me, I'd chew him out in front of the entire faculty meeting, and shame him into doing the right thing!"

"Your intentions are good," Mattie said, smiling, "But honestly, I'm glad you aren't representing me in this conflict. If I got in a shouting match with him in a faculty meeting, he'd be so irritated that he'd probably give me the worst assignment he could think of, and he might even try to get me transferred. Which is a polite way of saying fired."

"Where does he live?" Jane joked. "I bet he's not as tough as all that. I'll challenge him to a duel on his own front lawn. I bet you didn't know I was an expert swordswoman, did you?"

"It might be easier to master fencing than to become a conflict wizard," Mattie said, "but I think it wouldn't be quite as useful. I'm a teacher, not a pirate, after all."

"Okay, do it your way," Mattie said. "But at least make sure you do go and talk to him again."

"No more avoiding," Mattie said. "I promise."

7. TRANSFORMATION

When you use reflective listening to identify the true feelings and interests beneath the surface of a conflict, you reveal a puzzle you must solve. The puzzle is how to transform the situation so as to better satisfy everyone's underlying interests. It is a puzzle you must work on together. Only by cooperating can you find desirable solutions, because each of you holds some of the pieces of the puzzle.

The puzzle at the heart of the conflict is produced by the way your interests collided. The initial configuration is not a good fit. You've got to find another configuration that lets you pass each other without bumping. Or you've got to solve the puzzle by combining each of your pieces creatively to give you something new and better.

Have Your Looked Under Every Hat?

Once you've explored the root causes of the conflict and are looking at the pieces of your shared puzzle, your likelihood of success is directly related to how persistent and creative you are. Wizards know they can find good solutions to conflict puzzles by transforming them—if they try hard enough and explore enough options.

But coming up with creative new insights and ideas is not always an easy thing to do. For instance, if I said to you, "You have 60 seconds to come up with six good new ideas for products your business could sell," well, you would probably complain that it's not a fair question. So, how do we come up with good ideas and insights when we need them?

First, it is important to *study the problem*. We usually do not know a problem or other topic in as intimate detail as is needed for really good creative thinking. Then, once we have studied it, the next essential step in creative problem-solving is to *create a flow of ideas*. Not just one idea. Not just 60 seconds of thinking. But a real, on-going flow of ideas, over time and in their own time.

If a business wants to get some good ideas from its employees (say for saving costs or introducing new products or coming up with a better idea for an ad campaign), what does it do? The most traditional way—and it is time-honored because it works—is to set up a suggestion system. This system at a bare minimum consists of a visible box or place where ideas can be put, with some commitment to review them regularly and recognize or reward the best ones.

To solve a conflict or any other problem creatively and well, you need to set up a "virtual box" for ideas about it, and keep the box open for thoughts at all times. It is, really, just a corner of your mind which you are going to keep open for possibilities. Something you see, do or hear when not thinking about the problem might suggest an unexpected idea, and then you can add it to your mental box for later sorting and examination.

Applying the Problem-solving Formula

For someone like Mattie, the teacher who is trying to transform her conflict with her Principal, it is important to both study the problem in detail, and to stay open to ideas and thoughts until she has developed a real flow of them.

Mattie realized that she did not really have a full grasp of the Principal's issues and options. For one thing, it was hard to visualize all the possible ways of reassigning teachers to different classrooms. There are two classrooms or sections for most of the grades, each with a different teacher assigned to it. Mattie pulled out a pencil and piece of scratch paper from her purse and wrote down the list from memory. She stared at it for some time.

"You aren't a very good conversationalist," her friend Jane complained. Jane was driving; they were on their way back from a fun weekend trip to a music festival.

"Sorry," Mattie said, "I was just trying to get my mind around this problem of how to assign the teachers."

"Well, why don't you start with what you know?" Jane suggested. "Do you know which ones are going to stay on and teach next year?"

"I can guess pretty well," Mattie said. "Carlos, one of the second grade teachers, told me he had gotten a job offer in a school much nearer to his family, and was seriously considering it. I'll bet he is one of the ones the Principal is trying to find a replacement for."

"Did you say someone was getting fired?" Jane asked. "I love hearing about scandals, do you know who it is and why?"

"The only thing I can think of is that maybe the new fourth grade teacher didn't work out. I don't know her very well, she just came at the beginning of the year. One of my students has a younger brother in that class, and I gather from what he said that there were a lot of disciplinary problems and the teacher had trouble keeping the children organized."

"That's not much of a scandal," Jane complained. "I was hoping for a harassment case or a story about a teacher stealing school equipment or something exciting like that."

"Well, of course there was the teacher who kidnapped the principal's pet dog and held it for ransom, do you think he'll be fired?"

"Seriously?" Jane said, then realized that Mattie was teasing her. "Okay, never mind the scandal theory. But I bet you're right that if one of the fourth grade teachers wasn't effective, she might be replaced. So now you know, or at least can guess, that they need someone to step in and teach both a second grade section and a fourth grade section next year."

"Yes. And we also know that one of the new teachers the Principal is about to hire is only qualified to teach sixth grade. So I bet he's assuming I will have to take either the second or fourth grade class and give up my sixth grade class for the new teacher."

"And then he'll hire another teacher to cover the other class?" Jane said.

"Yes, I'm sure he will. But probably he can find someone qualified to teach it and not make things even more complicated. At least he didn't say anything to suggest there could be any other problems."

Jane thought for a minute. "So what's wrong with your teaching one of those classes, anyway?" she asked Mattie.

"Oh, nothing really, I guess, except that I haven't taught either of those grades before, so it would mean a lot of extra preparation work for me over the summer."

"And you're planning to go to school yourself this summer, aren't you?" Jane said. "Didn't you get a grant to study something?"

"Yes, I'm going to take a special class on teaching history. It's something I've been wanting to do for a long time."

"So, that's the only problem, the preparation for the class?"

Mattie laughed. "I wish you were my Principal, Jane," she said. "You are a lot more interested in my concerns than he is."

"I tell you, all I need is ten minutes alone with him and I'll have him begging for his life," Jane said. "Or I know what. Did I ever tell you about my Uncle Guido? He can be very persuasive, you know. Want me to give him a call?"

"Hold on," Mattie said. "No tough stuff! There's a solution here somewhere, I can smell it."

"We'll leave my Uncle Guido out of it for the moment, because maybe you don't want to owe him any favors," Jane continued. "But let me ask you this. Are there any other classes you 'd be happier to teach?"

I used to do a fifth grade class, and I get along really well with John, who teaches one of our fifth grade sections right now. I could probably handle the other section easily."

"Great, problem solved!" Jane said. "By the way, who teaches that other fifth grade section, the one you want to teach?"

"Oh, well, that's a potential problem too, actually. Angela has done it for a couple years and she probably wouldn't want to change any more than I do."

"That's okay, we'll have my Uncle Guido talk to Angela," Jane said. "By the way, has Angela taught a second or fourth grade class, so that switching to one of them might be easy for her? Not that Uncle Guido cares, of course."

"No, I don't think so," Mattie said. "Angela taught seventh grade before she switched to fifth. Which reminds me, there is a seventh grade teacher who used to teach second and first grades, and I remember him saying recently how he really missed working with the younger kids."

"Okay, so if you could get him to cover the second grade, then you could teach his seventh grade...no, wait, you said you wanted to teach fifth."

"But if Angela was interested in switching back to seventh grade again...hmm. As I remember it, I think she liked teaching the older kids but had to switch to fifth when we lost our fifth grade teacher a couple years ago. I might just ask her if she's interested in switching back."

"So let me get this straight. You are thinking that two other teachers might want to switch classes, and that if they did, it would free up a fifth grade class for you to teach, which would be easy for you to do. Right?"

"Right!" Mattie said. "I'll check with those other two teachers. If it's an I suspect, they will both welcome the chance to make the changes I suggest. Then we could all go to the Principal with our idea. Which would mean he could still put the new teacher in my sixth grade class, but I could switch to fifth which I already know how to handle. And the other teachers would trade around to get the classes they want most, too!"

"It's as good as solved," Jane agreed with her friend. "But what was that you were saying to me the other day about not wanting to give up your classroom?"

"Oh, that's another problem," Mattie said. "I get chilled easily and my sixth grade is in the warmest classroom right now. It wouldn't work to move fourth or second graders in there because we try to keep them clustered by age. But I wonder if the Principal would be willing to let me stay in my current room, and just change it from a sixth to a fifth grade room? The classes are right next door anyway, so it wouldn't really cause any problems for anyone."

"Wow, we're good!" Jane said, smiling. "We should hire ourselves out as creative problem-solvers. We might put my Uncle Guido out of business!"

"Do you really have an Uncle named Guido?" Mattie asked.

"As a matter of fact, I do. My Dad's family was Italian. His brother Guido is a famous painter, and also very active as a volunteer in his church. He doesn't bust many kneecaps, but I like dropping his name anyway. It sounds pretty tough, don't you think?"

"You're ridiculous, Jane. But I appreciate all your help. And I can't wait to run this idea by everyone when we get back. It seems like a real win-win to me."

A win-win-win-win, I think, and that's not even counting the new teacher who gets your sixth grade slot," Jane corrected. "Yup, this plan could potentially benefit you, the Principal, and several other teachers. Why wasn't it obvious from the beginning that this solution was possible?"

"I guess we overlook a lot of possibilities, if you think about it," Mattie said. "I wonder what else I should be thinking about. Have any ideas for how I can work things out better with my ex-husband?"

"Well, did I ever tell you about my Uncle Guido?" Jane said.

Transformative Magic

The secret to transforming conflict puzzles is to begin with an optimistic belief that you can. If you know there are always hidden alternatives to find, you won't give up too soon.

Then make sure you do your research, so that you have truly studied the problem with care and have plenty of knowledge about it. This usually requires use of reflective listening skills, since you will have to learn about the problem from the other people involved in the conflict.

Then you can open yourself up to a creative flow of ideas. Seek new ways to define the problem. New views lead to insights, which help generate new alternatives and options. It may take a little while, but if you open yourself up to the problem, you are likely to come up with some new ideas and approaches that could make it easier to meet everyone's needs.

Conflict wizards try to fight the circumstances, instead of the people. They seek new ideas that aid them in their struggle against limitations. They keep inviting new possibilities and suggesting alternatives long after others would have given up. They know that persistence is one of the easiest and most powerful tools to use in any kind of problem-solving.

Conflict Resolved

When Mattie followed this sequence of conflict-handling techniques and was truly persistent in her search for a better way, she did find a hidden solution that seemed likely to please all parties involved. So Mattie ran her idea by the other teachers, and found that they were in favor of her approach. They too had heard some rumors that they might be reassigned, and they much preferred to come up with their own plans than to be the victims of whatever plan the administration came up with. So, armed with her good ideas and her fellow teachers' support, Mattie set up another meeting with the Principal.

"Didn't I just see you a few days ago about this?" he said by way of opening. "I'm always happy to see you, Mattie, but I have to tell you that, honestly, I have not had time to make much progress on next year's schedule yet."

"Well, I think I have," Mattie said, smiling. "So this time, instead of putting you on the spot with more questions, I'd like to run an idea by you. Is that okay with you?"

"Okay, shoot," the Principle said, leaning back in his chair and grimacing as if in fear she really might shoot him.

Reading his defensive body language, she decided to work a little harder on opening the conversation before presenting her idea. She didn't want him to react to it with a quick, thoughtless "no" before he had a chance to really think about it and understand its merits. So instead, Mattie decided to revert to a little more reflective listening. She said, "I sense you're a bit defensive today, Jim. Has someone been in here before me who didn't have nice manners?"

"Your instinct is uncanny," the Principal said, grinning ruefully and relaxing a bit. "To be honest, I just had a rather difficult conversation with an employee who won't be coming back next year. I hate having to tell someone they are terminated. And she, I mean this employee, didn't take it very well. It's a long story and I don't intend to tell you it, but yes, I probably am a bit on the defensive right now."

"Well, you can relax, because this isn't something you have to give me an answer on right now. I just want to run an idea by you that may make next year's scheduling a lot easier on a number of us, including you."

"And I bet it makes things easier for you, right? Wait, don't tell me. I bet your idea involves your continuing to teach sixth grade." He smiled again, but she thought perhaps it was just a bit forced.

"No, as a matter of fact, it doesn't. I remembered what you said about the new teacher who you want to have teach my grade next year, and I decided to try to figure out a way to make things work out so that could happen."

"You're not leaving, are you?" he said, suddenly looking anxious. "Because that's not what I had in mind at all. You're one of our best..."

No, no, don't worry!" Mattie said, realizing that conflict communications were surprisingly difficult, even when you did have a better idea you wanted to share.

"Well, then, I don't see how we can avoid your having to cover one of the grades I'm losing teachers from," the Principal said.

"Which I'm guessing might be the second and fourth grades," Mattie said. He gave a slight nod. "But what if I told you that there was another teacher who has been hoping to get a chance to teach second grade again, and is eager to switch into that classroom next year?"

"But then I have to find someone to cover that teacher's..."

"I told you, Jim, all you have to do is sit back and listen!" Mattie kidded him. "Let me do the thinking for a minute here, and then you can decide if you like it or not. Because I happen to have yet another teacher, who wants to take that first teacher's class. And I happen to be eager to take the other teacher's class. So all I'm saying is that if we shuffle things around a bit, I think there is a way to move three of us around so that each of us would teach the class level that we are most comfortable and qualified to teach. Want to hear the specifics?"

"Really?" the Principal said, sitting forward and looking interested. "That would be great, but do you think the other teachers would agree? I don't want to make more problems while trying to solve this one."

"I've already talked to them," Mattie reassured him, "And they are happy to talk to you about it in person if you want to make sure it is all clear. I just didn't want to descend on you three-strong this morning without giving you fair warning."

"Thank you for being considerate of my nerves," he said. "That might have been intimidating coming right after my last meeting. But I'll talk to them later this week, before I draw up next year's schedule. It sounds like a winner to me, and thanks for working on the problem, Mattie. I really appreciate your taking such a constructive approach."

"My pleasure, and a benefit to all of us," Mattie explained. "But there is just one other thing."

"Ah," the Principal interrupted, "I bet I know what it is. The room, right? You want to stay in your room. I know you think the other rooms are too cold. But didn't you say you were going to take over one of the fifth grade classes? Why don't we just switch the signs on the doors, and let you stay where you are? The classrooms are the same size, and they are next door to each other anyway, so that shouldn't be a problem."

"That's a great idea!" Mattie said, perhaps a little over-enthusiastically, because the Principal looked at her quizzically for a second, then said, "You'd thought of that too, hadn't you? I bet you were just waiting to see if I figured it out, and if not, you were going to tell me that was the rest of the plan."

"Well, maybe," Mattie agreed with a laugh. "But you know what they say, Great minds think alike!"

As Mattie discovered, Conflict Wizards' good listening skills allow them to probe beneath the surface to identify the underlying interests or concerns. Then Wizards use creativity and persistence to transform the problem into a puzzle that can be solved in new and better ways. Finally, they break down the natural barriers to get the other party communicating with them openly enough to truly share ideas for problem resolution. Wizards put their energies toward transforming conflicts so that the impossible is often achieved, and everyone wins.

0. A CALL TO WANDS

*A*s we have seen through the experiences of Mattie, Conflict Wizards handle conflicts and disagreements very differently from other people. What exactly do they do different? The most important hallmarks of the Wizard's approach to conflict are these:

- Wizards find out exactly what everyone needs, taking more time and care than other people might to listen and explore. This helps them see the underlying interests, so that they do not get trapped into a fight over the positions people have taken. Positions and demands are just the surface of the conflict, where dragons breed and grow strong. Wizards seek to know the conflict's true nature by looking beneath the surface.

- Wizards insist on examining lots of alternatives, putting more time and care into looking for clever ways out that satisfy everyone's needs. They study the problem, then they generate a creative flow of ideas to help them solve it.

- Wizards avoid retaliation, knowing that attempts to "get even" are not truly cathartic and just fuel the fires of anger and misunderstanding, producing more and worse conflicts in the future. [14]

- Wizards avoid venting in ways that irritate others, knowing that the accumulation of minor irritants will make it far harder for the other person to collaborate with them in the future. [15] If people irritate a Wizard, he or she stops and applies reflective listening and fact-checking skills right away. The Conflict Wizard's motto is: Fix the little conflicts and you won't have big conflicts!

- Wizards never say they disagree with or oppose the other party, knowing that this frontal assault on the other person's position raises their defenses. Instead, Wizards explain why they disagree or why they cannot do something the other wants them to do. This subtle difference of approach reveals the Wizard's underlying reasons and interests, leading to a more open, collaborative approach and defusing the aggressive aspects of the conflict. *(16)*

• Wizards are soft on people, but hard on needs—which is just the opposite of most people's instinctive reaction in a conflict. Wizards avoid judging or criticizing or blaming the other party. Wizards know that people get upset and feel defensive, and that this makes people present their concerns in attacking ways. So Wizards don't pay attention to how others present their concerns. Instead, they insist on understanding those concerns. Wizards take a tough line on needs, not giving up until they have found reasonable ways to meet the underlying needs that caused the conflict of interest in the first place. *(17)*

When Wizards start by listening and reflecting the other person's underlying needs, then follow up with these other conflict-handling techniques, they are able to resolve conflicts effectively, and often in collaborative ways. They tame their conflict dragons with ease, harnessing the energy of conflicts for mutual benefit. Better communications allows these wizards to work through their conflicts more easily and effectively, and to help others with their conflicts as well.

Each Conflict Is Unique

Is every conflict handled in a win-win, collaborative manner? Not necessarily, but each conflict should be handled well. For instance, when Mattie went to buy a new-used car from the local auto dealership, she found herself negotiating with a tough, secretive salesman who was determined to get as high a price from her as possible. He ducked many of her questions and lied about the dealership's costs (she was pretty sure he was lying, anyway). She realized the dealership just wanted to get a good price for the car, period. So all she could do was put in a bid that she thought was at the bottom of their price range.

Her hunch must have been right, because the salesman at first said no, then agreed (at Mattie's urging) to think about it for a few days. When Mattie called him next week, the car had still not been sold, and

now he was more open to her low price. She eventually bought the car
for a hundred dollars more than the offer that he had rejected the previous week. (She thought the extra hundred was for him to save face,
so she left it on the table. It was only 1% of the price, so not really of
importance to her deal. And she really liked the car.)

In this experience of a more competitive negotiation, Mattie
found that her good conflict-handling skills were still useful. She
stayed calm, did her research, and asked a lot of questions, and she got
a much better price than she would have before she studied conflict
management. She did not really expect or need to develop a true collaboration with the salesman, but she did need to make a deal that
both of them could feel good about.

And Mattie's other conflicts improved over time too. She got better about not losing her temper with her ex-husband, for instance,
once she realized that she was in the habit of reacting angrily to certain triggers—and that he always pushed them when they talked.

At first, she talked only to herself (and her friend Jane) about this
pattern of behavior, and vowed to beak it. But even then, she found it
difficult. Some of the things he said still upset her. So she decided to
tell him about the problem too. After all, it was in his interest not to
have her so mad or upset they couldn't talk and plan on behalf of the
children. So in the end, he agreed not to say things like, "Why is it
always about you?" Mattie told him he was free to think that if he
wanted, but would he please refrain from saying it, since she just
couldn't stop herself from getting mad each time he did. And he
agreed to this, as it seemed a reasonable and minor compromise to
him. Communications went better after that, and in future years, they
sometimes even made jokes about it.

As for Mattie's relationship with her boss, it became more open
and trusting as a result of their successful collaboration, and they
often cooperated to solve problems in the future.

The Wizard's dance is very different from the destructive patterns
of the typical conflict. It goes something like this:

Recognize conflict situations.

**Manage your reactions to prevent instincts from taking over.
(Your understanding of conflict styles is very helpful here!)**

Reflect to identify underlying interests.

Shift the focus away from win-lose surface demands to new win-win approaches for serving the underlying needs.

Study the problem, then harness a flow of creative ideas to help redefine or transform it into a puzzle you can solve for mutual benefit.

Communicate to build consensus on a win-win solution to resolve the conflict optimally.

Sometimes the Conflict Wizard must gracefully bow out of this dance before it reaches completion, choosing to compromise or use one of the other conflict-handling styles if collaboration just isn't going to happen. Other times, the Conflict Wizard will sense that the conflict dragons are too powerful and nothing productive can come of the conflict, and will withdraw immediately to avoid destructive results. In still other situations, the Wizard may reflect upon the issues and decide that the other party's concerns are much more important—and then the Wizard will concede (accommodate) and give way gracefully to their demands.

In all of these different conflict-handling styles, the wizard's use of good listening and emotional management techniques keeps the channels open for reasonable and honest communications, whether about this conflict or the next.

But often, more often than you might think, the Conflict Wizard is able to reach a good solution that truly does involve a transformation of the problem and a collaboration with the other party to find a better way for everyone involved.

The music of this dance soothes the conflict dragons. It is a constructive approach that harnesses the dragons' energy and turns it to good.

Care to join the dance?

Epilogue

W e left you deep within a cave, face to face with a conflict dragon, sword in hand. What did you decide to do?

As an apprentice Wizard, you probably had the good sense to realize that the most important thing to do first was to decide what *not* to do! Whatever your natural conflict style might be in that situation, hopefully you had the presence of mind to interrupt that instinctive reaction and take charge of the conflict instead.

For instance, if you are a natural fighter, well, being cornered and threatened like that is going to make you see red. Your instinct is to come out fighting. But as soon as you take even one aggressive step with a conflict dragon, you can expect the dragon to escalate. And no matter how sharp your sword, escalation with a conflict dragon (or with just about anyone for that matter) can get messy in a hurry.

If you are naturally more peaceful and your instinct is to avoid or concede, well, you might feel an urge to give yourself up and throw yourself upon the mercy of the dragon. Again, not such a great instinctive reaction. The dragon might spare your life, but then again, it might just eat you up.

If you favor compromise, again your instinct would tend to leave you high and dry. You want to emerge from that cave with your life. Half a life won't do! And besides, the dragon seems to be in control right now, not you. How can you initiate a civilized compromise? Your instinct to compromise isn't going to get you out of this corner.

What if you are a collaborator by instinct? Many people are—in fact, the majority of people prefer to resolve most conflicts through collaborative, friendly problem-solving approaches. And as a collaborator, you probably realized right away that you might be able to use your sword to untangle the rope that is giving this disgruntled dragon its toothache.

Hold on. Wait a second! You thought the solution to the mystery of the conflict dragon was to recognize that the dragon had a toothache and to trade your dental services for your life? Well, that is a good insight, to be sure, and you certainly need insight. But it's not quite that simple.

Look at it from the dragon's perspective. Even if it hopes you will help, how will it know that it can trust you? As soon as you start mucking around in its mouth with a sharp sword, it may get scared and toast you to a crisp or nip your arm off. Trust is a difficult thing to create in the tense context of a conflict. It takes care and sympathetic communication to set the stage for a collaboration.

So, the first thing your wizard training should have taught you is to do none of the things that your instincts first urge upon you.

Instead, your wizard training should have taught you to engage the magic of reflective listening as your first step.

It is always necessary to open and invite if you want to take control of a conflict—or a conflict dragon.

Once you establish open communication with the dragon, then you can clarify all the underlying interests. Clarifying means exploring the dragon's needs, not just leaping to a quick conclusion.

You may simply find as you suspected that the dragon is bothered by the rope and would like to remove it. But until you and the dragon get that out in the open through reflective listening, the dragon will not know that you care. It will not be able to trust you with its problem until you've worked the magic of reflective listening.

But how do you listen to a dragon? Does it even speak your language? Will it even know that you care? Hmmm. Too bad you haven't taken that upper-level dragon-lore seminar yet, or you might know more about this predicament.

But one thing you do know for sure: You won't be able to communicate with this dragon unless you try. So let's get started.

How You Save The Day
(and save your neck in the bargain)

The head now looms above you, the gnarled jaws open, and you find yourself staring at its glimmering fangs, barbed tongue, and glowing throat. Suppressing your instinct to lash out and then try to run, you inspect the dragon's teeth closely, focusing on the tangle of rope around several of its fangs. You clear your mind and try to focus on how it is feeling, then talk quietly to it, trying to mirror those feeling, to let it know you understand.

You start by saying something like, "Hmm, oh dear, that looks painful. Does it hurt? That rope is tangled all around your teeth. Is it bothering you? It must be uncomfortable. Are you okay?"

As your soothing, sympathetic words fill the silence of the dragon's cave, the red glow in the back of its throat dies down and it lets out a low moan that seems to confirm your diagnosis. Then its long, barbed tongue licks one of the fangs and wiggles it.

Puzzled, you examine the tooth the dragon has just touched. The rope is wrapped all around it. You say, "Is the rope hurting this tooth in particular? Should I take the rope off? Want me to try to cut the rope away?"

The dragon snorts and shakes its great head, nearly knocking you over. You realize you must not have fully appreciated its situation, and so you reexamine the tooth. It is certainly wrapped with rope. But the dragon seemed to have said that the rope wasn't the problem after all.

But if not the rope, what then? Maybe the dragon misunderstood you. You decide to try to clarify the question once more, saying in as soothing and sympathetic a tone as you can, "Isn't this rope bothering you? It is tangled all around that tooth. It sure looks to me like the rope is the problem."

But again, the dragon shakes its head. Then it turns to one side and emits a sudden roar of flame and smoke. When it turns back toward you and opens its mouth, you see that the rope is burned completely away. Only a few smoking threads remain in the dragon's mouth. Which means, of course, that the rope was not the dragon's problem.

You are feeling confused. If the dragon could remove the rope that easily, then why had it permitted the rope to stay there in the first place?

You decide you had better try to communicate your confusion about the dragon's underlying needs. You say, "I can tell that something is bothering you, Dragon, and I'd like to help, but I just don't know what you want. What is it? What do you want me to do?"

Now the dragon wiggles that fang with its tongue again, and this time, with the rope gone, you can see that the tooth in question is in fact surprisingly loose. Not only that, but it seems to be more yellowed than the other teeth. It must be old or rotten!

The dragon has a bad tooth, you realize, so you try out this new insight, saying, "Oh, I see! Your tooth is rotten. It is almost ready to fall out. It must be sore. It's a bad tooth, right? And I bet you were trying to remove it by using that rope to pull it out. Is that right?"

Now the dragon nods its head up and down, as if to agree with you. At last you understand the dragon's true underlying interest! Now maybe you can try to help out. You say, "I could probably get a good grip on it with my hands and pull it out. Should I do that?"

The dragon nods in the affirmative.

But before you try, you realize you are not in a very good position to be doing dental work on dragons. You are still feeling very vulnerable and concerned for your safety, and the cave is becoming intolerably hot as well. So you decide to try to communicate your own feelings to the dragon. "I think I can pull that tooth out, but it's going to be a tough job and I'm feeling pretty weak and frightened right now, and if I get any hotter I'll probably faint. Would you mind if we went back out to the mouth of the cave?"

The dragon stares at you unblinking for a long while, then finally seems to decide you are trustworthy and backs away, leaving a path open for your escape.

You climb carefully back over the pile of treasure, putting the sword back down where you picked it up and saying "I don't think we'll need this," then walking calmly back to where you had deserted your belongings when the dragon first surprised you.

You slowly pick up your stuff and return it to your pack, setting the pack by the door in readiness for your departure. Then you beckon the dragon nearer and roll up your sleeves in preparation for the operation.

It comes up to you, opens its mouth, and closes its eyes as if preparing for a painful experience. You reach in slowly, grasp the rotten fang in both hands, and try pulling it toward you. It rocks forward, almost coming out, but seems to be stuck, and the dragon winces and pulls back. Now what?

You decide to ask the dragon. "Do you want me to pull harder? It's going to hurt, but I think it will come out if I really pull it as hard as I can." The dragon nods yes, then presents its mouth again, and this time you grab the yellowed fang and give it as hard a jerk as you can.

And now the tooth breaks off in your hands, pulling free of the coral-red gum and falling with a clatter onto the stone floor.

The dragon licks the opening where the tooth had been, and you notice that there is the sparkling tip of a new tooth pushing up to take the old one's place. The dragon leans down to sniff the tooth, and noses it toward you along the floor. You pick it up and add it to your pack of belongings.

Finally, the dragon bows its head low before you as if to say thanks. You return the bow. Then, turning, it crawls back into the rear of the cave, leaving you alone at the entrance.

The rain has stopped and a full moon appears from behind a retreating cloud, illuminating the door of the cave and the path beyond it. You shoulder your pack once more, pick up your wand, adjust your robe and hood, and head back out to complete your journey. Later, when you have time to speak to one of your professors, you'll ask what the significance of the gift of that tooth is. Perhaps a dragon's tooth has some magical properties, or maybe it is just a token of appreciation for your collaborative approach. It will be interesting to find out.

∼

Don't forget to praise yourself
when you succeed.
It takes plenty of reinforcement
to modify our own conflict behaviors.

∼

The Workshop

~

Wizard Workshops
Real magic for real people who want to
master the things that matter most

~

~ The Wizard's Workshop ~

*I*n this section of the book, you'll find a selection of some of the most powerful and intriguing activities and tools from our conflict-handling, teamwork, communications and negotiation workshops.

- If you are using *Taming the Conflict Dragon* in the context of an organized workshop, your workshop leader or instructor will guide you to the specific activities to do first. And you may be given advance reading/doing assignments so as to make your time together in the seminar or meeting as productive as possible. (It will, of course, help if you actually *do* these advance assignments. Thanks!)

- If you are reading this book for your own pleasure and advancement, you can benefit from the same exercises used in professional seminars by sharpening your pencil and doing these activities on your own. Each of them comes with enough instructions and information for you to do them independently. Let the Conflict Wizard be your teacher as you participate in these "virtual workshops" to hone your skills.

By the way, each of these interactive learning modules provides backup and depth to one or more of the chapters in the Conflict Dragon Guidebook you have (presumably) just read:

Workshop 1. Understanding Your Conflict Style

The workshop materials start with a section on exploring your own conflict style, which gives you a way to go deeper on an important topic that first came up in Chapter 2, *Finding the Dragons in Your Life.*

Assigned? _____

Completed? _____

Workshop 2. Flexibility Defeats the Dragon

In Flexibility Defeats the Dragon, you'll see how to adjust your approach to make sure you are using an appropriate style for each disagreement, conflict or negotiation you encounter.

Assigned? _____

Completed? _____

Workshop 3. Helpful Strategies for Emotional Management

Here the wizard gives you some practical tools of relevance to Chapter 5, Taking Emotional Control of the Conflict.

Assigned? _____

Completed? _____

Workshop 4. Avoiding Emotional Words and Other Red Flags

Next comes a module on red flags, which you'll find very interesting as you learn more about the topic of Chapter 5 and go even deeper into the challenge of taking emotional control. Conflict dragons can slip in and steal control whenever people fail to manage the verbal and nonverbal cues in a conflict, so the exercises in this section are among the most powerful of any we've ever included in a workshop or course.

Assigned? _____

Completed? _____

Workshop 5. Playing Collaborative Games

This is an interesting activity in which you get to explore the competitive nature of most of the games we play in our formative years, and then try your hand at a new version of an old game in which the only way to win is to overcome competitive instincts and share your thoughts and insights to solve a puzzle together. (Perhaps you noticed that this is just what the wizard in the story had to do to solve his problem and escape without having his beard singed off.)

Assigned? _____

Completed? _____

Workshop 6. Finding Reasonable Criteria

In all conflicts, it is helpful to agree on reasonable criteria for use in discussing possible solutions. In fact, discussing decision-making criteria can often help reduce tensions and improve communications to de-escalate a conflict.

Assigned? _____

Completed? _____

Workshop 7. An Ounce of Prevention

You'll find in this wrap-up to the Wizard Workshop a short hands-on section concerning how to try to detect early warning signs of potential violence in the workplace. As the introduction to the book pointed out, while most conflicts do not lead to violence or injury, there is always the slim possibility, and so it is only prudent to be aware of trouble and try to head it off. An ounce of prevention is worth a pound of cure, as the Conflict Wizard likes to say.

Assigned? _____

Completed? _____

Each of these sections is based on an activity from a training program or product that we have used many times with groups of adult learners (and sometimes in classroom settings with younger learners as well). Here you will find them converted to entertaining self-study versions that you can pursue on your own initiative, or do as preparation for a short discussion session or meeting with others from your workplace.

Learning can be a wonderful adventure, especially when it is about a subject as vital as conflict-handling skills. Enjoy this novel way of taking a Wizard Workshop!

∼

W1. Understanding Your Conflict Style

*E*ach person has a style or pattern of behavior when put under the pressure of a conflict situation. This style can differ from one person to another. But whatever your particular style is, you need to understand it fully before you can handle conflict well.

In this section of the book, you can take a simple survey to find out what your instinctive responses to conflict are and explore your own style.

Why explore your own style? They say that self-awareness is the root of all learning. This is doubly true when it comes to learning skills that involve elements of human behavior. For instance, someone who reacts angrily to challenges will always be the victim of her own temper, unless she learns to recognize and change this pattern of behavior. In professional as well as in personal life, success is often dependent upon our ability to understand and manage our own behavioral responses.

Here is an example of how an understanding of style helped someone handle conflict better, allowing him to advance in his career.

Joshua Learns Not to Give In Too Quickly

Joshua was recently promoted to be the head of a sales team representing complex medical equipment. His new duties include negotiating sales and service contracts with doctors and hospital administrators for the equipment his company makes and sells. Many of these orders are customized to meet the specific needs and preferences of the hospital in question, so the contracts can vary from one sale to another.

Joshua recently took a survey to assess his conflict style, and learned that he tends to try to accommodate the needs of others. He is a "people person" who does not like the other people in a conflict to be angry or unhappy, and so he will often "go the extra mile" to solve their problems. He always builds strong, friendly relationships with the customers and they view him as helpful and concerned. In fact, this is why he was promoted to head the team.

Knowing this, however, Joshua is careful to control himself when customers press for unreasonable demands, and to ask for time to consider their requests. He does not want to let his instincts take over and give away too much when negotiating a contract.

Often Joshua finds that he is dealing with multiple people at a hospital—doctors from several departments, a senior executive, someone from purchasing, and perhaps even the legal department may be involved. And often, each of them has their own concerns and demands. When Joshua lets his agreeable nature take control, he has a tendency to promise all of them everything they want—even though it is not realistic or profitable to do so. Because his self-assessment helped him be aware of this tendency, he reminds himself to have "difficult conversations" in which he explains why some of their demands are unrealistic. He has become a better negotiator, and has avoided signing contracts that would only "come back to bite him" when unrealistic promises in them proved difficult to keep. Joshua is glad he understands his first reaction to such requests, because it keeps him from agreeing to something he will later regret.

Would you like to explore your own reactions to conflict? To do so, follow the instructions and answer the questions starting on the following page.

Take the Test: What Is Your Conflict Style?

Instructions: Decide how well or poorly each of the statements below applies to your behavior in conflict situations (focus on workplace situations if you are using this instrument for work training). Circle a number between 1 and 5 to show how well each statement describes your behavior:

Scale		
	1	definitely not
	2	probably not
	3	maybe
	4	probably
	5	definitely

---

1. I will fight hard to protect my interests.   1 2 3 4 5

2. I talk about what we have in common as a way of solving conflicts.   1 2 3 4 5

3. I prefer "splitting the difference" in order to avoid lengthy negotiations.   1 2 3 4 5

4. I much prefer a friendly discussion instead of a disagreement.   1 2 3 4 5

5. If I can stay out of an unpleasant situation I do.   1 2 3 4 5

6. When I have the upper hand, I use it to get what I need.   1 2 3 4 5

7. I am skilled at turning conflict into cooperative problem solving.   1 2 3 4 5

8. I often propose a middle ground that is fair to both sides.   1 2 3 4 5

---

9. My priority is to stay on good terms with people.

1 2 3 4 5

10. I don't like to confront others with my complaints.

1 2 3 4 5

11. I don't mind a good argument if it gets me what I need.

1 2 3 4 5

12. I like to share my feelings fully, and I encourage others to do so too.   1 2 3 4 5

13. I'm happy to go half way as long as the other party does too.   1 2 3 4 5

14. In disagreements and conflicts, I want the other person to be happy with me by the end.   1 2 3 4 5

15. I do not feel confident about my negotiating skills.

1 2 3 4 5

16. I try not to reveal too much, for fear it may be used against me.   1 2 3 4 5

17. I see disagreements as opportunities to find a new way to solve our problems.   1 2 3 4 5

18. I don't waste time in lengthy discussions when a simple compromise is possible.   1 2 3 4 5

19. I will give in on issues in order to "keep the peace" in a disagreement.   1 2 3 4 5

20. When I think someone has an issue with me I try to stay out of his/her way.   1 2 3 4 5

21. I may use a threat or bluff when dealing with someone who is not being cooperative.   1 2 3 4 5

22. I expect honesty and trust on both sides of a discussion.

1 2 3 4 5

23. The most efficient thing to do in most disagreements is to split the difference.   1 2 3 4 5

24. I sometimes let other people win an argument if it makes them happy.   1 2 3 4 5

25. My opinion is that in many cases there is little to be gained by arguing or negotiating.   1 2 3 4 5

Please use the scoring form below to analyze your results.

Interpreting Your Answers

Please enter the number you circled for each question in the blanks below. (For example, if you circled 3 for question #1, enter a 3 in the first blank). Work from left to right.

After you have entered all your scores, add each column and enter each total in the box at the bottom of the column.

1		2		3		4		5	
6		7		8		9		10	
11		12		13		14		15	
16		17		18		19		20	
21		22		23		24		25	
Totals:									

   Compete   Collaborate   Compromise   Accommodate   Avoid

Each of the "totals" boxes is labeled underneath with the style it represents. For example, the first column (on the left) is labeled "Compete." You should have a score of anywhere from 5 to 25 for each of these five styles. Some scores will be higher, indicating that you generally favor those styles over others.

Often, one style is clearly higher than all the others. That indicates a preference for that style. Do you have a dominant or preferred style you usually use?

Other times, two or even three styles may be tied, indicating mixed preferences and a more flexible approach. If you have a tie, then you may alternate between two preferred styles, or you may tend to use one first, and then shift to the other if things aren't going well. Whatever your pattern, it is important to be aware of this tendency to use a single style or a style sequence in most conflict situations.

Which style(s) received the highest score when you took the test?

Preferred Negotiating Style(s): _____

This is the style you are most likely to use in conflict situations. But is it always the best style to use? Maybe not. Remember that you have many choices at all times during conflicts. Also remember that how well you use your preferred style or any style depends upon your ability to stay calm and in control of your emotions.

(Note: The questions in this test are similar to a technical tool we publish for assessing conflict styles, called the Dealing with Conflict Instrument or DWCI (available from TrainingActivities.com or from HRD Press). If you are participating in a course that uses the DWCI, then you do not need to take the above test too. You can simply use the results from the DWCI.)

Using the Styles Correctly

Here are descriptions of when and how to use each of these styles. Each has its proper place in any conflict wizard's repertoire.

ACCOMMODATE
(Be unassertive & be highly cooperative.)

Give in so they can win. Use this style when you want to make the other party happy and don't care about other outcomes. To use this style, simply let the other party know you are willing to give up your interests in the conflict so they can pursue theirs.

AVOID
(Be unassertive & be uncooperative.)

Refuse to address the conflict. Use this style when you don't want to deal with the conflict at all. Stay away from the other party, or if that is not possible, tell them clearly that you are not willing or able to deal with the conflict right now. They may not like this because then they cannot deal with it either, so be firm.

COMPROMISE
(Be moderately assertive & be somewhat cooperative.)

Find a fair middle ground. Use this style when you and the other party both want to deal with a conflict quickly and easily using the rules of compromise. To use this style, split your differences in even, fair ways.

COMPETE
(Be highly assertive & be uncooperative.)

Get more out of the conflict than the other party does. Use this style when you care more about the outcome than the relationship and are determined to win at the other party's expense. Also use this style when you are sure the other party is competing, and collaboration does not seem possible. To compcte, make demands that you know are more than the other party will give. Push them to offer concessions, and try to offer smaller concessions in return. If you compete effectively, you should reach agreement at a point that is more favorable to you than a straight compromise would have been.

COLLABORATE
(Be highly assertive & highly cooperative.)

Work together to redefine the conflict so both parties can win. Use this style when you can manage to break down the conflict barriers and get the other party to open up and work with you. Try to understand their perspective and try to help them understand yours. Be clear about what your concerns and desires are in the conflict, and find out what theirs are too. Then work together to seek many alternatives. The more options you consider, and the more creative those options, the more likely you are to find a way for both of you to come out ahead.

If you follow the above instructions when you use your preferred, natural style (the one with the highest score on the test), you will have more luck with it. "If it's worth doing, it's worth doing well," as the old saying goes!

However, you also need to practice using less-familiar styles, since there are times when your preferred style will not be as appropriate as another style. You may have noticed in the descriptions of each style (above) that there were some tips on when and why to use it. This is because:

**Each style has its role, but no one style
will handle all conflicts well.**

∽

For instance, when negotiating to buy a car, you may want to use the compete style effectively since the salesperson will probably be doing the same thing too. But, when discussing team assignments with a group of people you work with regularly, you may want to avoid a competitive approach. Competition won't work if you want to make sure the project gets done well. A competitive style would aim to do the least work and make teammates do the most. That obviously is not good for the project, or for the future of the team.

Teamwork is not a competitive game, so the compete style is inappropriate. The collaborate style is best. If you are a natural user of the collaborate style, you can just follow your instincts. But if you are a natural competitor, compromisor, avoider or accommodator, then a team project demands that you adapt your style. You have to learn some new tricks, even if you feel like an "old dog," and so it is helpful to study the descriptions of your alternate styles carefully (see above).

What happens when someone's natural style is inappropriate for the situation? Then their behavior in the conflict tends to be counter-productive. It opens the door and invites the conflict dragon in. Soon everyone is getting frustrated, tempers begin to fray, and the participants in this conflict find themselves dancing with the conflict dragon again. Too bad, but all too common—and simply because most people are not conscious of their own conflict style, and don't adjust it when the situation requires a different style instead. That's why the next section, *Flexibility Defeats the Dragon*, is a popular part of our conflict workshops too.

W2. Flexibility Defeats the Dragon

Conflicts escalate when one or more parties stick stubbornly to their own behaviors.

If you find that a conflict is getting worse as you try to compete (for example), then continuing to compete, or competing even harder, will not help. Yet that is most people's first reaction. Our style preferences become stronger when we are subjected to stress. So if we tend to be competitors, we will compete harder as the conflict gets worse.

Same with any of the styles. Someone who is a natural collaborator will try to reach out and engage a competitive salesperson in collaborative discussions. If this doesn't seem to be working because the salesperson is an aggressive negotiator, the collaborative customer will often try even harder to collaborate. The customer may share more and more information with the salesperson, since laying your cards on the table is part of a good collaboration. But sharing can only hurt the customer in this case, because the salesperson will use his information to strike a tougher bargain.

For instance, if the customer reveals that she really likes a special color and this dealership is the only one to have a car of that color in stock, guess what? The price has just gone up because now the salesperson knows this customer will not want to walk away. To get a fair price, the customer must recognize that the situation demands a competitive style, not the collaboration she prefers. This customer must be careful to hold her cards close to her chest until she has seen a firm offer she can accept. Otherwise, she is not likely to get a fair price.

The lesson is simple, but often hard to follow:
Whatever your preferred style,
if it's not working, *you have to stop!*

Some wit once defined insanity as "doing the same thing over and over, and expecting to get different results." It truly is crazy to keep using a conflict-handling style if it is not working well. The more you use it, the worse things are going to get, and the more likely you are to find yourself dealing with a conflict dragon—an out-of-control situation that is probably going to make you unhappy, if not cost you dearly, before it is all over.

So use your test results and your understanding of conflict style to recognize your own style. And be willing and ready to change it if the situation demands. Flexibility defeats the conflict dragon. Rigidity and habitual behavior fuel the dragon's fires.

Flexing Your Style in Response to the Situation

Sometimes it is helpful to use a simple but powerful rule of thumb for choosing the right style.

The rule of thumb is this:

Your style should reflect both your concern for the bone, *and* your concern for the other dog in the fight.

Well, OK, you are not actually a dog and you don't usually fight over bones. But your conflicts are with someone else, and they are over something you both want or need, albeit not usually a bone. So, to help you select the best style to use, decide how you truly feel about the other party, and about the "bone" (the thing you want to get or don't want to lose in this conflict).

Let's go back to that slippery car salesman who has the only car in the color our collaborative buyer likes. Now, the buyer's "bone" in this conflict is the car of her choice. She definitely cares about it. She wants a good outcome. She wants to be able to buy this car for a price she can afford and will feel good about later on.

What about "the other dog in the fight," the car salesman? Does our buyer care about her relationship to this salesman? Does the deal she gets have great importance to him, and is this a legitimate concern of the buyer? Not really. In fact, it's just another deal to the salesman. She need not worry about him, he can take care of himself. In fact, she can be quite sure he won't do anything that puts his commission or job at risk.

If he tries to enlist her sympathy with tales of a mean boss and tight economic times, she can be sure he is just playing his games and seeing what he can get from her. She has no obligation to take care of this salesman. The "other dog" is not an important concern when negotiating to buy a car. Only the car and its price are important in this conflict. That is why the compete style is appropriate and no other one will do. Buying a car is truly a competitive game, and the right thing to concern yourself with is getting a good car at a fair price.

But let's look at another situation. Imagine you are having a disagreement with your significant other over where to go on a long weekend.

If you hope to continue to be each others' significant others, then this situation is very different. Your concerns include not only having a good trip, but (perhaps even more important), having a good life together. If you play the tough, competitive negotiator in this situation, you will probably find yourself going to your favorite place alone. *(Sometimes the dog finds it is not happy all by itself, even if it has the bone.)*

So, the rule of thumb is to make sure you pick a style that is appropriate, given your feelings toward the other party, *and* your feelings about the subject or outcome of the conflict:

- If you only care about the outcome, go ahead and compete. But be careful not to let competition get out of control or you may get burned! Anger or hurt feelings call for a change of style immediately. They are never good outcomes.

- If you only care about the other person, then accommodate by letting them take the bone for themselves. Make it clear you want them to be happy and are giving them a gift. Sometimes it is best to invest in the relationship instead of fighting over the bone!

- If you are concerned about both sides of the conflict equation, then you better collaborate. Collaboration means working on both parties' concerns at the same time, so as to try to make both of you happy with the outcome. It is the only way to deal with the situation if you really need that bone—but also care enough about the other dog that you would never want to bite it.

- What if you care a bit about this conflict and the other person's interests in it, but you don't view the thing as worthy of too much time and effort? Try compromising. It is a quick, ritualized way to split the difference and let everyone get on with their lives. It may not be optimal, but it is easy and that is sometimes the priority.

• A final option is that the situation is not productive. Then you should avoid the conflict, even if means hiding under your desk until the other person goes away! If someone is just itching for a fight, walk away and give them time to cool off. It's amazing how many conflicts are all dragon and no substance. Avoid these like the plague—or like you would a dragon.

Sometimes in conflict workshops, we draw a grid to use in evaluating a situation or case and selecting the most appropriate strategy:

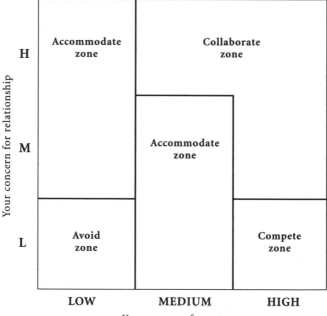

Wizards are "Closet Collaborators"

As the grid indicates, there is no one best style and your behavior needs to be flexible to defeat the conflict dragon. But along with this flexibility, conflict wizards do have a bias toward one style: collaboration.

That's why, in Chapter 7 of the book, it says that "the puzzle is how to transform the situation so as to better satisfy everyone's underlying interests." This collaborative problem-solving approach is powerful magic, and conflict wizards look for opportunities to use it. In fact, they never let an opportunity go by without testing to see if there is some chance to redefine the problem and achieve a breakthrough. Conflict wizards have this collaborative bias because they find that:

There are often hidden opportunities to collaborate.

∼

You may have noticed, in the grid used for choosing a style, that the collaboration zone takes up the largest area. There are many contexts in which collaboration works well. Not all of them are obvious, unless you are a conflict wizard. The conflict wizard is an inventive problem-solver who uses a creative problem-solving approach in conflicts, and this approach leads the wizard to see win-win opportunities where others do not.

Creativity is often defined as a way of thinking. But first and foremost, it is a way of *seeing*. You can't engage in creative problem-solving until you see the opportunity to do so. You won't think to explore alternatives unless you first recognize the possibility for alternatives.

How can you "see" better than others and uncover hidden opportunities to collaborate? By using your wizard skills to take emotional control and avoid escalation. And by being a good listener who "clarifies the reflection" using exploratory questions. Perhaps most important, your conflict eye-sight will benefit from stepping away from your own concerns and remembering to focus first on what the other person in the conflict is concerned about. In Chapter 7, the wizard's approach is defined as,

Listen first. Listen fully. Build understanding.

∼

There is plenty of time to assert your interests (if in hindsight they still seem important), *after* you understand the other party's interests more fully. Listen first. Talk later. It's a simple rule with great power to reveal opportunities for the two (or more) of you to do some joint problem-solving that avoids either of you having to give in. So remember to use your wizard skills to explore for hidden opportunities to collaborate.

All human progress is the result of a creative rejection of limitations. Who says humans can't make fire, build bridges, fly, cure diseases, or go to the moon? And if we can overcome such fundamental barriers to our human development, we can certainly overcome many of the more mundane barriers that arise as we try to work with other people and organizations in our daily lives.

(The Collaboration Game that appears later in this workshop section of the book is a fun way to practice creative problem-solving with another person. Dig out some old domino tiles so you are prepared to use them in this unusual game.)

W3. Helpful Strategies for Emotional Management

Your ability to handle conflicts and use any of the five conflict-handling styles well depends in part on how good you are at keeping your head in conflict and using some general strategies that work for any style. These strategies include the following sure-fire dragon-slaying techniques no conflict wizard would ever be without:

- ✔ Understand the other party's point of view
- ✔ Understand the problem clearly
- ✔ Avoid irritants to keep the other party cool
- ✔ Stay cool yourself
- ✔ Reach out to break down barriers and build empathy and cooperation
- ✔ Take a creative approach to the conflict

When you do these things well in conflicts, the conflicts will be resolved more easily and quickly, and both you and the other party are far more likely to feel that your needs are met.

Also, when you do these things in conflicts, you will find that the conflicts *do not escalate*. Escalation is when the conflict takes on more emotional and/or practical importance over time and becomes too complex and difficult to deal with.

Often simple, minor conflicts escalate into major ones. When this happens, emotions run high and it is very hard to resolve the conflicts productively. Destructive conflict handling behaviors emerge. The parties attempt to hurt each other. And in the long run, everyone loses (except that unwelcome conflict dragon, who thrives on destructive conflict behavior). In such situations, the parties often lose much more than was initially at risk before the conflict escalated.

So it is helpful to study and practice strategies for keeping conflicts under good emotional control. Here is a quick guide to how to use some of the most powerful of these strategies.

The first strategy is to understand the other party's point of view, something that is often harder in practice than it sounds in print.

Strategy #1
Understand the other party's point of view.

TACTICS:

Ask open-ended questions...
like "Why?" and "What are your concerns?"

Check your understanding...
by saying things like, "It sounds like you are worried about
_____. Is that true?"

Clarify/reflect their understanding...
by repeating what they say and asking them if that is exactly
what they are concerned about or if they meant something else.

When you make an effort to understand the other party's point of view, conflicts become much easier to understand and handle.

The next strategy is to explore the problem itself and make sure you understand it as clearly as possible. Often we enter into conflicts with strong opinions about what we want, but without a full understanding of the conflict itself or how we got into it.

Strategy #2
Understand the problem clearly.

TACTICS:

Explore their thinking...
by analyzing their concerns and asking for more information.

Share information incrementally.
Offer information about your own issues, and ask for information in return. Build up a pattern of information exchange by showing you can be trusted to respect their concerns.

The third strategy is to try not to upset or anger the other party. Often, we accidentally escalate conflicts by triggering emotional responses. For instance, imagine someone says to you, "Since you're getting angry, don't you think that we should postpone this discussion?" Will you calm down or get more upset when the other party says this? Usually such comments make people mad. This quote includes two classic irritants: it tells you how you are feeling ("you're getting angry") and it tells you what you are thinking ("don't you think that...").

Strategy #3
Avoid irritants to keep the other party cool.

Don't tell them what they think or how they feel.
Ask them what they think and feel.

Don't tell them how they are behaving.
(Also called labeling.) If they are "being a jerk," telling them won't help. Instead, model better behavior yourself. (A related tactic is, Don't tell them what they are trying to do. Ask them what their intentions and motives are.)

Don't praise yourself.
Saying things like "I'm making a generous offer" or "I'm playing fair, so why don't you?" always irritates the other party.

Don't defend yourself.
The other party may say or do something to hurt you. If you retaliate, you are starting a defense/attack spiral. They will attack back. And the conflict will escalate. Withdraw or if you can stay calm, ask them why they are attacking and what their real issue is. But ignore the attack!

Do use open, friendly body language.
Much of what we say is nonverbal. If you keep tapping your foot impatiently, saying "I'm listening, what's on your mind?" won't do any good. It's obvious (to the other person) that you don't really want to listen to them. Be careful to "square up" so you are facing the other person rather than seeming to avoid them.

Make polite eye contact so they know you are listening. Try to signal your interest and openness by smiling and nodding.

Remind yourself to avoid typical defensive postures that arise when we feel stressed (don't cross your arms, rear back, or frown). These defensive nonverbal responses generate the same sorts of nonverbal behavior in the other person. And when the nonverbal signals start to escalate, the language and thoughts tend to follow.

Anger and other strong emotions like feeling hurt, embarrassed or challenged are the enemies of good conflict management. But it's hard not to get emotionally involved and "heated up" by a conflict. If this is tough for you (it is for everyone I've ever met), then you might want to take a look at the later section of this book in which we look more deeply at emotional words and other "red flags" and how to avoid them.

The fourth strategy involves staying cool yourself so you can manage the conflict well and help the other party stay cool too.

Strategy #4
Stay cool yourself *(even if they don't).*

TACTICS:
Focus on the long term.
Remind yourself of where the conflict started and where you want it to end. This will help keep you from going down a side path.

Take breaks…
whenever you feel yourself becoming emotional.

Watch yourself.
Imagine you are watching your own behavior from a distance (maybe you're on a hidden TV camera!). How are you behaving?

Are you using your conflict-handling skills or forgetting them? Do you need a break to calm down and get in control?

Understand the reasons for their behavior.
Ask yourself what they are doing that irritates or upsets you, and why they are doing it. When you understand the reasons for their behavior, it won't make you as angry.

Breaking down barriers is a related strategy, because it can only be used when emotions are calm:

Strategy #5
Reach out and break down barriers to build empathy and cooperation.

TACTICS:
Show consideration by asking how they feel, or offering to do something to make them more comfortable.
Showing that you care about them, even when you disagree with them, is a very powerful strategy!

Make conciliatory gestures.
Concessions, even very minor ones, often help improve the feelings between parties in a conflict. And if you make a series of small, even symbolic, concessions, eventually the other party will begin to reciprocate. Then you can move on to more meaningful concessions and begin to problem-solve productively with them.

Be willing to apologize.
It's amazing how powerful a simple apology can be. It is like the proverbial "oil on troubled waters," soothing feelings and smoothing the pool of collective emotions.

Apologies are appropriate whenever your actions have upset the other party—whether you feel you were logically "in the wrong" or not. You can be sincerely sorry you upset, hurt, irritated or inconvenienced someone, even if you think you had a right to say or do what you did. So don't overlook this simplest and most ancient of conflict-handling techniques. An apology shows you care how the other person feels, and caring is a very powerful thing indeed.

Once you reach out and begin to lower the barriers, it is possible to shift to a more creative problem-solving style. The ideal is to get the other party to collaborate with you in finding a new and better way of handling the conflict.

Strategy #6
Take a creative approach to the conflict

Find out exactly what everyone needs.
Explain your needs more specifically, and probe to explore their needs fully too. Often a new and better solution is easy to see once both parties understand their needs fully. When you share concerns and needs, you set the stage for creative problem solving.

Insist on examining lots of alternatives.
Most conflicts involve two competing alternatives, one favored by each of the parties. When you make the effort to develop at least a few more alternatives, often one of them proves appealing to both parties and the conflict evaporates.

Activity: Observing a Conflict Communication

Here is an activity you can do to explore and deepen your awareness and understanding of these powerful strategies. The basic idea of this activity is to analyze any conflict by observing one of the people closely while they communicate. As an observer, you concentrate on seeing if they use some of the strategies.

What conflict can you observe? If you are doing this on your own as a reader, you could keep the activity in mind while watching a movie at home. Movies often have rich examples of conflict communications. If you find a good one in a movie you like, try following one of the characters and using the checklist below to observe whether the character is employing these strategies and tactics:

☐ Asked open-ended questions?
☐ Checked his/her understanding?
☐ Clarified/reflected the other party's understanding?
   ☐ = **Understood the other party's point of view**

☐ Explored the other party's thinking?
☐ Shared information incrementally?
   ☐ = **Understood the problem clearly**

☐ Didn't tell them what they think or how they feel?
☐ Didn't tell them how they are behaving?
☐ Didn't praise one's self?
☐ Didn't defend one's self?
☐ Used open, friendly body language?
   ☐ = **Avoided irritants to keep the other party cool**

☐ Focused on the long term?
☐ Took breaks?
☐ Watched him/her self?
☐ Understood the reasons for other party's behavior?
   ☐ = **Stayed cool**

☐ Showed consideration?
☐ Made conciliatory gestures?
☐ Was willing to apologize?
   ☐ = **Broke down barriers to cooperate**

☐ Studied everyone's needs?
☐ Examined lots of alternatives?
   ☐ = **Took a creative approach?**

> ؛ریرى

W4. Recognizing Red Flags

*I*t usually seems as if people are arguing about the substance of a disagreement, but if you listen more closely, most arguments are not so much about what people say as how they say it.

Conflict dragons love to take advantage of the ways we communicate in conflict. They feed on the nuances of word choice, tone of voice, gesture and other things that can act as "red flags" to upset or anger us or others.

In workshops, we often ask two people to play the roles of co-workers who are having a disagreement about their contributions to a team project. The two roles are scripted as follows. Imagine two different people are reading the parts for A and B, or find someone to help you read them out loud.

A. "Um, hi, listen, I wanted to ask you about that last team meeting. Did you really mean what you said about your department not being willing to cooperate on reports any more?"

B. "Now hold on a minute, I think you're over-reacting and you certainly did in the meeting. I got a lot of flack for that later and all I meant was that we have to balance the reports with the new assignments we were given after the downsizing. We've got our own problems and it doesn't help for you to get mad about this."

A. "Nobody's mad! I'm just trying to find out what you meant, because if we can't count on you any more, we need to know about it right away."

B. "Of course you can count on us, you're always trying to make it sound like the problems are at our end. But it seems like your department is usually late with the information we need to do the report in the first place."

A. "Now hold on one minute! That only happened once and you know it. The real problem is that the information sits in your inbox for two weeks before anybody ever touches it. If it's too much for you to handle, why don't you just tell us and I'm sure we can get somebody else to take your place on the team."

This conversation has a natural tendency to escalate into a heated argument. What would "B" say next? Probably something that "A" will feel is not very nice, to say the least. But what might a conflict wizard do? Is there a better way to handle this discussion?

Thinking About What We Say, And HOW WE SAY IT

Whenever people read these parts out loud, they tend to "ham it up" like actors, and they grow increasingly upset with each other.

Why does this happen? What is it about the script that signals an argument instead of a friendly problem-solving session?

The answer is emotional words. Some words and phrases have a strong, negative emotional impact, and should be avoided in conflict situations. These emotionally-charged words can act as "red flags" that distract the other person from the substance and generate a defensive emotional reaction.

As the wizard taught us in the guide-book, in conflicts, both parties usually believe they are defending and the other person is attacking. And, of course, escalation seems justified if it is in self-defense. Why do people feel they are being attacked? Because red flags signal an attack—even if one was not intended. Red flags can be nonverbal as well as verbal. Here is a table listing some of the most common red flags, including emotional words, labeling of the other person's behavior, and nonverbal actions/reactions that also tend to generate defensive responses.

"RED FLAGS" THAT FUEL DEFENSIVE SPIRALS

Wording ⇓	Tone of Voice ⇓	Body Language ⇓
"Always"	Angry	Too close, "in face"
"Never"	Condescending	Pointing finger, offensive
"You"	Manipulative	Too distant, not attending
"Why are you…"	Put upon, whiney	Hands on hips, tapping toe, impatient
"You should…"	Judgmental, certain	Defensive postures, crossed arms or legs
"Don't be…"	Cross-examining	Frowning; angry eyes
"Be serious"	Too loud	Raised eyebrows, disapproving
Uncooperative	Disgusted, fed up	Not smiling
Angry	Speaking over other person	Not making open eye contact
Declarative (vs. questioning)	Raising volume toward end of sentence	Not squaring up to listen respectfully

Red flags like these can easily interfere with your efforts to reach out and communicate with someone in a conflict. If they use any of these red flags, your own conflict dragon may see the flash of red and come racing in to raise the temperature even further. If you accidentally use some of them on someone else, the other person's dragon may be attracted to the flag and make them act angrily or defensively.

Often, people are puzzled as to why a conflict seems to have gotten out of hand. The comment, "What did I say?" expresses this surprise. The answer may not be so much what we say, as how we say it. By avoiding red flags and trying to ignore them when others use them, we can keep focused on the substance and not allow the conflict dragons in.

Recalling Your Own "Red Flags"

Here is a related activity you might want to try. Think about times when someone "attacked you" in a conflict by behaving in a way that made you uncomfortable, upset, angry or defensive in response. What specific things did they say that upset you? It is amazing how the emotional words are often easy to recall, even if we can't quote the rest of what they said. Emotional words are felt more than heard, they can sting or burn, and so we recall them somewhere deep down where conflict dragons hide. Bringing them out in the light of day can help stop them from having power over us.

Try making a list of specific words or phrases someone used that you did not like or that upset you in recent conflicts:

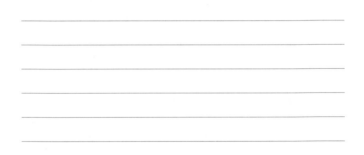

Now think about the nonverbal behavior that might have accompanied these emotionally charged words. Were there other signals or actions that also stick in your emotional memory? Did the person, for example, tend to interrupt you or appear not to be listening to you?

Try to list some examples of nonverbal red flags that may have bothered you in conflicts you have experienced:

Good work! By surfacing these red flags where you can see them, you can reduce their power to call in the conflict dragons. Some people even try things like writing their worst red flags, the things that really upset them, on an erasable board and then ERASING THEM to symbolically erase the power they hold over us. Whatever your approach, make sure you realize what is going on when you next hear or see a red flag, so that you can remind yourself not to give it power over your emotional response to conflict. And please try not to wave red flags in front of others, unless you really do want to call in the conflict dragons. It's ever so much easier to summon a dragon than to send one away.

THE ANGER MANAGEMENT FORMULA SAYS THAT:

Seeing + understanding
the causes of our angry or upset reactions
keeps us from losing emotional control.

Break the cycle with your knowledge of emotional words and other red flags.

~

W5. Playing Collaborative Games

*L*et me ask you a question that often proves challenging in our workshops on conflict-handling skills:

**Can you make a list of a dozen or more
truly collaborative games people play?**

By collaborative, I mean non-competitive, where the object is not to win by making someone else lose, but rather to win together. Win-win games instead of win-lose games. And by game, I mean broadly, any fun activity people play both to entertain and to develop their skills.

Baseball and chess are both examples of games. However, they are not collaborative games since their goal is for one side to beat the other.

Ah, I bet I know what you are thinking! You are saying, isn't baseball collaborative since you work together with your team? Yes, as a team sport, it is more collaborative than chess which you play alone. But baseball is not completely collaborative, since it aims to produce a win-lose outcome, not a win-win outcome. Playing with the goal of a tie every time would be stupid. It's an inherently competitive game, and the competition is a good part of what makes it exciting and interesting to play or watch.

That's fine, I'm not knocking baseball. But because its fundamental premise is to win at the other team's expense, it is in its own way teaching competitive conflict-handling, not cooperation and teamwork. The same basic attitude that leads to a win in baseball might also be found in a tough, competitive labor-management negotiation over a new contract. Each side works together to beat the other. They do not share their strategies or plays, or even talk much to the other side, since they are competing. As a result, they are not going to solve any tough problems or make any significant strategic improvements to the business upon which they all depend. All they can do is argue over their respective slices of the existing pie. It takes collaboration to bake any new pies, metaphorically speaking.

If you want to generate a cooperative atmosphere in a family or workplace, competitive games are not the best models. The experiences we gain playing them are not directly relevant, and in fact may lead to counterproductive behaviors. (We certainly can't have people acting in their offices they way they do on the sidelines of their child's Little League games!)

That's why we seek examples of fully collaborative games, ones in which people work together for a win-win solution. Are there such games? Do we have examples we can use as models? Are there games we can play to practice our collaborative skills? When we ask this question in workshops, it quickly becomes apparent that there is a competitive tradition in our society, and that most games reflect this tradition. They are fun, but they are not always good models for how we want our co-workers, bosses, employees, spouses, or children to behave.

So, let's go back to that opening question. Have you come up with any examples of truly collaborative games in which the participants engage in a quest for a win-win outcome?

Kind of hard, isn't it?

Here is one example. Girls sometimes skip rope together, teaching each other new patterns and chants to go with them, and even holding the rope for each other. Jump rope is usually a collaborative game, where the artistry of the achievement is the goal.

Hacky sack is another collaborative game. Have you seen young men keeping a soft little bean-bag ball in the air by standing in a circle and kicking or kneeing the ball to each other like arm-free jugglers? A group of three to five people can keep this difficult game going for minutes at a time.

How about board games or card games? Hmm. Not many of those are collaborative. The only one that comes to mind is Owija, an "occult" game in which everyone puts a finger on a gliding piece that then is moved mysteriously around a game-board, touching letters to spell out messages from the "spirits" in answer to participants' questions.

Some of the building-block-oriented children's toys support cooperative play. For instance, children may work together to see how tall a tower they can build out of blocks or how elaborate a bridge or spaceship they can make out of Legos.

My children used to play an interesting collaborative game with a big sheet of drawing paper and a large bag of color pens. Each person would start drawing in one corner of the page. Then, after an agreed-upon time of several minutes or so, they would rotate the page and start adding to or working on the corner the person to their right had started. With enough rotations to fill the page, they would have made a truly collaborative drawing that tended to take fascinating creative turns none of them would have thought of on their own.

Although my kids probably didn't know or care, this drawing game is in a way a variant of a writing game invented by French artists in the previous century, and called The Exquisite Corpse. You fold a piece of paper so that it has three sections, then write a single word in the first. Next, fold your word out of sight and pass it, second section up, to the next person who writes another word, then refolds it and passes it for a third person to complete. You are collaborating "blind" in that you don't have any idea what the other two people are writing, so it is entertaining to see what you get. The very first time it was played, the three words were (as I bet you have by now guessed) "the exquisite corpse," hence the name for this unusual collaborative game.

These are varied examples of collaboration in our play, and they prove that it certainly does occur, even though it is rarer than competition.

Let's play!

If you can put your hands on a box of domino tiles (the most common sets have 28 pieces or tiles), then all you need is a co-conspirator who would like to sit down across the table from you and learn a new version of this old-fashioned game.

The traditional dominos games all work on the assumption that you want to beat the other players. We are going to modify the rules so that the only way to win is to work together. Follow these steps to set up:

1. Divide the tiles into two equal piles, keeping them upside down (so you can't see the number of dots on each half of each tile).

2. Each player sets aside 8 upside-down pieces, to form his or her BANK. It will be drawn on later if the player doesn't

have a move from his hand   see step 3

3. Each player turns over 6 pieces to form his or her HAND.

4. Prepare to play by making sure you understand the rules of placing tiles and scoring a round.

5. Play a round, total your scores, enter them in a log or table, and then turn over (upside down) and shuffle the pieces in preparation for the next round.

Tiles are placed in dominos by matching like-numbered ends. A tile with three dots on one end can be matched to another with three dots—but only on the three-dot ends. Tiles are placed end to end (long ways) unless you run out of room in the playing area, in which case you can make the line of tiles take a 45 degree turn.

You can only work from open ends—where someone hasn't already placed a tile.

Some tiles have the same number of dots on each end of them. They are "doubles" and are played cross-wise instead of length-wise. They form two open ends instead of just one.

Players take turns moving.

When you lay tiles down according to these rules, sometimes you find you have an open end to which you can match one of the pieces in your hand. If not, then you have to take pieces from your bank until you either find a match or run out of pieces. When a player cannot move (runs out of pieces in his/her hand, or runs out of bank pieces without getting a match), then the round is over. Score the round by counting how many pieces you have in BOTH your banks, minus the number left in BOTH your hands. The goal is to have full banks (16 pieces between you) at the end of the round. Use a table like this to score the rounds:

Round	Total number of pieces in both of your banks	Minus total number of pieces in both of your hands	Equals combined score for the round
1		−	=
2		−	=
3		−	=
4		−	=
5		−	=
6		−	=
7		−	=
8		−	=

At first, most players get a few moves into a round, then get stuck and have to start taking pieces out of their banks. See if you can find a way to play this game so as to protect the pieces in both your banks and emerge with high scores of 15 or 16. It can almost always be done—if you play the pieces you've both been dealt in the optimal order! But how will you do that? First, you'll have to decide what your strategy is and how you want to approach the problem together, with a shared plan. Then you can decide who goes first and what to do at each step.

What Changes When We Play Collaborative Games?

In playing the cooperative dominoes game (which is marketed by TrainingActivities.com under the name *Cooperation!*), you find that your approach to play changes with experience. At first, you will probably play fairly quietly, each thinking independently about their next move. This is typical of competitive games, which is why they don't prepare us well for true teamwork or group projects and problems.

With a bit more experience, most players begin to communicate much more. They share ideas and questions, and discuss their two hands at length before either makes a move.

And when they are playing, they begin to seek agreement before moving, instead of just moving their own pieces and then waiting to see what the other player does.

Another change is visible when players encounter a problem—when they anticipate that they may get stuck, or one of them actually does run out of moves. At first, they tend to stew on these problems individually. Only with several rounds of experience do they learn to talk them through together. When they communicate more fully about problems, they generally are better at finding solutions that don't cost as many points.

As a result of these shifts from traditional competitive-play behaviors to collaborative-play behaviors, pairs of players usually find that their scores improve. The scores in the opening rounds may be fairly low. Scores get higher as the behaviors change.

This game is fun to play simply because of the challenge of solving each new set of hands and trying to get a high score. It is also intriguing because of what it teaches us about our natural competitive-play habits, learned from many years of playing more competitive games.

We find our communication and decision-making habits changing in order to collaborate more effectively in pursuit of the common goal. The game illustrates the profound differences between competitive and collaborative styles of conflict management, and gives us some clues as to why it is often hard for people to adopt truly collaborative approaches, even when they wish to do so. Until they practice those new, collaborative communication and decision-making behaviors, their old habits may continue to get in the way.

~

W6. Finding Reasonable Criteria

"I want X."

"Well, I want Y."

"I'm sorry, but Y is totally unacceptable.
We really have to have X."

"Actually, Y would be a major problem from my perspective.
I'm not clear on how you even came up with it."

"Well, to us, X seems unreasonable.
We've never used X in a deal like this before."

*H*ow is this discussion progressing? Are they going to resolve it anytime soon? Probably not, because they have not stopped to think about what criteria there are using and whether they are reasonable. If they did, they might be able to agree that, say, W was the most common and generally acceptable criterion for the decision. This might lead them both to switch to W and find it acceptable.

In this module of the Wizard's Workshop on Conflict, we will switch from the focus we have had on the "soft" aspects of conflict handling: things like your personal style, your interpersonal skills as you avoid "red flag" words and actions and use reflective listening. These aspects of conflict handling are very important, but sometimes the "hard" aspects of how you structure the conflict and its solution are equally important.

In fact, in the previous activity, you probably found it necessary to combine sound thinking and strategies with good communications to solve the collaborative puzzles posed by your need to empty your hands of domino tiles. Hard and soft elements combine in any conflict. It takes clear thinking as well as open communications to solve most conflicts. And the criteria you use to define the possible solutions are part of the way you think about the conflict, and need to be given careful consideration. Often it is necessary to agree on the criteria you will use, before you can achieve any breakthroughs in the conflict.

The Power of Reasonable Criteria

Imagine a buyer and seller are haggling over price. If they both have knowledge of what fair market value is, they are far more likely to come to agreeable terms efficiently. That's because:

Fair market value is a reasonable criterion in many cases. The Blue Book publication gives average sale prices for used automobiles in the U.S., and is often used in transactions as a point of reference when used cars are bought and sold by private individuals. Without this reasonable criterion to go by, sellers and buyers would lack confidence and find it difficult to know a good deal from a bad one.

Equal treatment is another reasonable criterion. For instance, if two parties have to find a way to divide something, they might agree that it was reasonable to split the thing in half so as to give each an equal amount. Compromises work because of the reasonableness of equal treatment. Another way to divide things fairly is for one person to do the dividing and the other to do the choosing. That way the person doing the dividing has a strong incentive to do it fairly.

Custom is often seen as a reasonable criterion too. If there is a clear precedent or tradition, the parties can refer to it for guidance. They might do some research or ask someone with more experience than them what the customary approach is in their situation. As long as the custom seems reasonable, it will probably be acceptable to both sides. This approach is used to set royalty rates when intellectual property (inventions, writings, artistic creations) are bought and sold. For instance, publishers customarily give authors between 10% and 15% of net sales on a hardcover book. Any author trying to negotiate for a rate higher than this customary range risks being seen as unreasonable.

Reasonable criteria switch the focus away from *what* each party demands and toward a discussion of *how*. That is a useful approach in many conflicts. Dragons like to fight over who gets what. They are repelled by rational discussions of how a decision should be made.

COMMONLY USED CRITERIA

- Potential market value
- Cost structure/reasonable margins
- Investment/appropriate return on investment

- Expert opinion
- Fair division/equality
- Sharing of risk
- Time spent/time investment to date
- Fair market value
- Customary practices
- Taking turns
- Establishing who was first
- Deciding what is ethical
- Deciding what is legal

Activity: Finding Reasonable Criteria

In the following cases, see if you can suggest reasonable criteria that both parties are likely to find acceptable. If you can find a partner or small group to do this activity with, it will be easier to make quick progress. You should discuss each situation and consider the possible criteria, then choose one that is most likely to seem reasonable and be acceptable to both parties.

Case #1

Two nurses are arguing about who should have to cover a shift on a popular holiday. Each complains that they have had to work on holidays too often in the past, and each wants to be with their family for this holiday. But one of them has to work, since the shift must be covered. What reasonable criteria would you suggest they use in deciding this issue?

What criterion is most likely to seem fair and reasonable to both parties in Case #1? How would you advise the nurses to resolve their dilemma?

Case #2

The core group of employees of a start-up company are upset because the owner and founder has just announced the sale of the company. Under the terms of sale, the owner will get $1.5 million in cash and another $3 million in stock options, and the company will become a wholly owned subsidiary of the public company that is acquiring it. But the employees say the payment and options should be divided equally among them, not given only to the founder. They claim that the founder did not pay them fair market wages, and that they had a verbal agreement that they were going to be given equal shares of the company's equity. However, before they got around to formalizing this arrangement, the owner got an unexpected buyout offer and sold the firm without consulting them. These employees feel cheated and are threatening to try to hold up the sale in court. What reasonable criteria would you suggest the various interested parties use in deciding this issue?

What criterion is most likely to seem fair and reasonable to both parties in Case #2? Can you think of a good way to banish the conflict dragons that are circling over this startup company and threatening to cheat it of its success?

Case #3

A team of employees was charged with redesigning the work flow in an office to make sure that paperwork is handled more efficiently and accurately. They volunteered to join the team, even though it required extra work without additional compensation. At the time they signed up, their managers explained that it was a high-profile assignment that would most likely be rewarded with fast-track promotions later on.

When the team studied the work flow in their department, they realized that it had many unnecessary steps. Their report recommended computerizing most of those steps and reducing the number of people involved by half.

When management read the report it embraced the proposals and immediately downsized the department. To their surprise, all of the team members' jobs were eliminated and they were given two weeks notice. They approached management and demanded the promotions they felt they had been promised, but were turned down flat. Their senior managers say business is poor and they need to cut the payroll. The employees are considering hiring a lawyer and pursuing their claim in court, but management would like to avoid a legal battle. What reasonable criteria would you suggest they use in deciding this issue?

What criterion is most likely to seem fair and reasonable to both parties in Case #3? Can you head off what looks like an ugly labor-management dispute and keep the conflict dragons from dragging the argument into court?

Case #4

A manufacturer met a sales representative at a trade show and the sales rep expressed strong interest in one of the manufacturer's newest products. Eager to test the market, the manufacturer agreed to let the rep try to sell the product for a month on a trial basis. The manufacturer gave the rep specification sheets, price lists, and samples. They discussed terms and the rep said a 20% commission was customary. The two shook hands on it and went their separate ways.

A few weeks later, the rep submitted a large number of big orders, surprising the manufacturer. In fact, the manufacturer had to scramble to scale up and produce these orders and ended up losing money on them as a result.

When the manufacturer called the rep to find out what was going on, the rep demanded immediate payment of the 20% commission, explaining that she had devoted herself to launching the new product to the exclusion of everything else and needed the money to cover expenses.

The manufacturer responded by arguing that they had only discussed testing the product, not going all out to write so many orders so quickly, and questioned whether the orders were of high quality. He said that he couldn't pay the rep her commission right away because he wanted to wait and make sure there weren't returns or uncollectables. He proposed paying the commission only on the good orders, 90 days out.

The rep accused the manufacturer of going back on his word and said, "I knew I shouldn't have trusted you without a written contract." (Notice that "emotional words" are creeping into this conflict!)

The manufacturer took offense at being called untrustworthy, and the conversation ended with him slamming down the phone.

What reasonable criteria would you suggest they use in deciding this issue?

What criterion is most likely to seem fair and reasonable to both parties in Case #4? Can you help them find a way to work together, since obviously the sales rep is capable of helping the manufacturer achieve a high level of success if they can find a way to collaborate?

116

Suggested Solutions

Case #1

The two nurses may both have reason to complain that they get stuck covering holiday shifts more often than they want to. It sounds as if there is no existing system in place for allocating this chore fairly. Perhaps they could agree to divide these shifts evenly among the staff in the future, rotating through them in sequence so that they can anticipate when they will or won't have to be on duty far in advance and make their holiday plans accordingly. Fair treatment is most likely to be seen as a reasonable criterion in this case.

But even if they agree to rotate holiday shifts in the future, who will "start" by covering this one? They could agree to flip a coin to see who goes first, as this is generally considered a fair criterion since it gives each an equal chance. Or they could conceivably agree to go back through the records and see who has covered the most holiday shifts in the past, and give that person this holiday off. That method would also appeal to their sense of reasonableness. In fact, it might seem more reasonable than flipping a coin if one or both of them feel there has not been a fair division in the past.

Did you come up with one or more of these ideas yourself? Or do you perhaps have an even better idea for resolving the nurses' dilemma?

Case #2

The owner might dispute the employees' claim, pointing out that there is no written evidence to support it (and indeed the employees were naïve not to have obtained something in writing!). On the other hand, the combined word of the employees and any evidence they can put forth showing they were paid below normal market rates might be enough to at least raise the possibility of an implied contract—and therefore hold up the sale while legal wrangling goes on. If the sale is made complicated enough by this dispute, the acquiring company might well back out and then nobody would profit. So they need to establish some reasonable criteria and reach a negotiated settlement quickly. They might look for precedents from similar cases as a reasonable criterion. Or they might ask an arbitrator or other expert for an opinion. A third solution is that they could possibly make reference to standard salary levels, using them as a criterion for deciding how much the employees were underpaid and asking the owner to make up the difference now.

Case #3

The employees have reasonable grounds to feel mistreated, since they were not treated the way they were led to believe they would be. They might favor criteria such as ethical treatment, keeping one's word, or following up on commitments. On the other hand, management might reasonably be able to show that conditions have changed and would therefore argue that they have the right to make whatever decisions are necessary for the good of the company—another potentially reasonable criterion, but not one the employees are likely to agree with.

Since the two sides have far-distant positions and no obvious common interests (aside from avoiding a messy legal dispute), it is probably best to seek a fair-division compromise. Each side could estimate what they stand to lose (and each will probably agree that the likely value of the salaries in question is a reasonable starting point for discussions). They could reach some sort of settlement that represents a fraction or multiple of each employee's annual salary.

Alternatively, they might explore the legal issues and find out to what extent the verbal representations to the employees constitute a contractual obligation. An objective legal opinion might be a good criterion for starting their negotiations.

This is a very tough case—maybe you noticed! With good conflict-handling skills and a commitment to good communications, a situation like this need not have occurred in the first place. Yet read the business section of any major newspaper and you will see conflicts of this sort happen all the time. Your ability to identify reasonable criteria can help you use your wizard skills to defuse the situation and keep the conflict dragons from taking control.

Case #4

Both the manufacturer and sales rep have the potential to profit from their relationship, since the new product is a runaway success. (That makes this case a classic for the use of a collaborate style.) But until they agree on reasonable criteria and clarify their terms, they will be unable to move forward and profit from their relationship.

In this case, the best approach is to use cash flow needs as the key criterion. Both are worried about their cash positions and need to protect their businesses from short-term losses in order to be able to afford to move forward and profit from their relationship. So the best criterion is what each needs in order to successfully fill orders and launch the product. If they come around to the same side of the table and work out a practical plan, then allocate their cash or other needed resources as necessary to implement it, they are more likely to achieve business success. Otherwise, they will waste their efforts arguing and fail to do profitable business together.

Lessons Learned?

In all of these cases, the parties involved are initially quite far apart and are going to have trouble finding a zone of agreement unless they can first agree on some reasonable criteria.

By asking the question, "What are the most reasonable criteria to use in this conflict?," we shift the focus from who is right to how we can find a fair and acceptable solution.

You may have noticed that some of these cases were best handled collaboratively, because the participants had to continue to work together and so would benefit from making sure everyone is happy with the outcome, not just one side. (Those nurses in Case #1 may work together for years to come. We don't want either of them to feel bad about the outcome.) In other cases, the solution need not be as collaborative. The managers and employees in Case #3 will probably go their separate ways. But regardless of which style is best, the solution of every case requires that the parties agree on reasonable criteria. Reasonable criteria, like good listening skills and a careful avoidance of red flags, are universally useful, regardless of what style you choose to use. Wizards realize that:

**Without reasonable criteria, no two parties
will ever agree on a solution.**

~

~

W7. An Ounce of Prevention

Wise wizards know that sometimes conflict can turn ugly, when people bottle up resentments or frustrations and then act out their anger physically. A spouse may throw things or strike a loved one, and in the workplace, people sometimes vandalize things, steal, or even attack others. These events are rare, and there is no reason to think that disagreements and conflicts will inevitably turn violent. Most do not. However, in any workplace (where we do most of our workshops), it is important to be aware of the possibility that someone may act out their anger in an unacceptable or dangerous manner.

The old saying that an ounce of prevention is worth a pound of cure certainly applies to the threat of violence in the workplace.

Can we prevent workplace violence? Probably. Most incidents that get reported in the papers are perpetrated by someone who, in hindsight, people say they were concerned about or expected to do something bad. Well, then why the heck were they allowed to have free access to that workplace? How come nobody did anything to help the perpetrator or prevent the violence from occurring? Usually it turns out that people did not think they were responsible for preventing potential problems. And often, they did not feel comfortable raising the alarm. So it makes sense to think about what you would do if you saw any warning signs in your workplace. Do you know what to do? Who to call? And most important, do you know what warning signs to look for?

Most people have a fair idea of what to do if they think there might be a problem. They can talk to their human resource department, building security, their boss, or the police. So why don't they? Because they don't know what warning signs to look for. When they get an uneasy feeling, they tend to dismiss it, not realizing that they may be seeing signs that have been indicators of violence in past incidents in workplaces like their own.

So here is a checklist that attempts to formalize the identification of warning signs and makes it easier to discuss or report anything that makes you nervous or concerned. Use it to evaluate your workplace periodically. In fact, why not start right now? (And please feel free to reproduce or modify it. We view this as a work in process.)

VIOLENCE PREVENTION CHECKLIST

In your workplace,

1. Has anyone said threatening things toward others?
    ☐ no   ☐ yes*
2. Does anyone feel angry about being mistreated?
    ☐ no   ☐ yes
3. Do people have access to guns?
    ☐ no   ☐ yes
4. Has anyone said they want to get even with their boss or
    the organization's management as a whole?
    ☐ no   ☐ yes*
5. Do people sometimes feel afraid of others?
    ☐ no   ☐ yes
6. Do people sometimes express their anger physically?
    ☐ no   ☐ yes
7. Do people sometimes lose control of their tempers?
    ☐ no   ☐ yes
8. Do people fail to report suspicious behavior on the part of others?
    ☐ no   ☐ yes
9. Do people fail to report threats made by others?
    ☐ no   ☐ yes*
10. Do people not know who to speak to when they are concerned
    that someone might behave violently?
    ☐ no   ☐ yes
11. Do people ignore someone who is angry or threatening?
    ☐ no   ☐ yes*
12. Are there any individuals who have acted irrationally and
    strangely in the past?
    ☐ no   ☐ yes
13. Are there any individuals who seem to "have a chip on their
    shoulder?"
    ☐ no   ☐ yes
14. Is there anyone who people think is likely to "go crazy one day?"
    ☐ no   ☐ yes
15. Are there people who nobody knows?
    ☐ no   ☐ yes

16. Are there people who live alone without any close personal relationships or emotional support?
    ☐ no   ☐ yes

17. Do some people feel that their treatment is very unfair or unjust?
    ☐ no   ☐ yes

18. Do some people feel like nobody ever listens to them?
    ☐ no   ☐ yes

19. Do some people feel like they are not at all respected?
    ☐ no   ☐ yes

20. Is there anyone whose habits and behaviors have recently changed significantly for no clear reason?
    ☐ no   ☐ yes*

21. Is there anyone who has behaved in a verbally abusive manner toward others?
    ☐ no   ☐ yes*

22. Is there anyone who has behaved in a physically abusive manner toward others?
    ☐ no   ☐ yes*

23. Is there anyone who has not been screened for past criminal activities and/or who is known to have a criminal record?
    ☐ no   ☐ yes

24. Are some people deeply depressed?
    ☐ no   ☐ yes

25. Do some people drink or use drugs to excess?
    ☐ no   ☐ yes

26. Do some people like to talk about violent activities?
    ☐ no   ☐ yes*

27. Do some people talk inappropriately about guns or explosives?
    ☐ no   ☐ yes*

28. Does anyone joke about violent things they are going to do?
    ☐ no   ☐ yes*

29. Do people often joke about violent things they expect someone else to do?
    ☐ no   ☐ yes*

30. Do you feel afraid for your safety or security?
    ☐ no   ☐ yes*

Any "yes" answer could deserve attention and follow-up action.

And if there are multiple "yes" answers, immediate action is definitely required. The Violence Awareness Checklist was compiled from risk factors identified by experts and from after-the-fact accounts of violent incidents in workplaces and schools. In most cases, several of these risk factors were present before a violent incident, but were not attended to. Only in hindsight did people realize they should have pursued the risk factor by asking questions, seeking help, or reporting their observations or concerns to someone who could take further action.

For example, listen to some of the newspaper accounts from interviews with people who knew the student who shot fifteen people at the Santana High School on March 14, 2001:

> "<Person 1> said the youth railed to him on Saturday night about wanting to shoot people, "But I didn't think he was serious. It's going to be with me for a long time...I could have done something about it.'"

> "Fifteen-year-old <Person 2> told reporters the suspect told him and others about planning a school shooting, 'but we thought he was joking. We're like, Yeah, right.'"

> "On Friday, <Person 3> said, "Williams nonchalantly said 'maybe I'll go to school on Monday and bring a gun,' but 'I didn't take him seriously.'"

> —All quotes from *San Francisco Chronicle,* 3/6/01, p. A4

If you have any reason to suspect or worry that someone might possibly behave violently, it is worth pursuing. You can take a variety of actions, including:

• Asking them how they are doing, if they are okay, or if there is any truth to the rumor that they are contemplating violence. Surprisingly, a common thread among many people who have behaved violently at work or at school is that no one spent time asking them about their situation or demonstrating interest and concern.

123

- Sharing your concerns with others and comparing notes, then taking action based on what you learn.

- Passing your concerns on to someone in authority who agrees to take action.

- Increasing security measures to make it more difficult to bring weapons into the workplace.

- Involving mediators, counselors or other professionals by sharing your concerns and asking them to get in touch with the person in question.

- Improving communications and conflict management practices throughout your group or organization.

- Remedying underlying causes of anger such as improper or unfair treatment or practices.

- Giving disgruntled or other at-risk employees more information and options so that they feel they can take non-violent action to improve their situation.

- Securing the workplace so that threatening people do not have access to it.

What if your concerns are unwarranted? Don't worry. You need not accuse someone of something they have not yet done. Just express your concern for them and refer to this checklist as your reason for acting.

You don't need to be sure to be concerned. If there are any reasons for concern, they are worth taking action on. Maybe your concerns are about someone who would never do anything violent, even if they had numerous and serious provocations. But there is no harm in showing concern—and if something bad did happen, you would never forgive yourself for not acting in time. When the potential risk is great, then it is reasonable to be safe rather than sorry, and people will (hopefully!) understand your desire to "err on the side of caution" as the old expression goes.

WARNING: Yes answers marked with "*" are sometimes short-term warning signs. Act on them immediately.

Putting the Activity Into Perspective

The vast majority of conflicts do not result in violence. And a significant share of conflicts are valuable and productive, if handled with skill and care. In living and working together, people often find their interests collide with those of others. To make progress in their lives—and to help their families, employers, and societies make progress as a whole—people need to acknowledge these healthy conflicts and use their skills to resolve them well. In other words, conflict does not automatically mean danger or risk of violence. Many conflicts are healthy and should not be feared or avoided.

And when good conflict-handling skills are used in a family, workplace or any other arena of human endeavor, people feel that they are listened to and that their concerns are resolved fairly. A sense of *fair process*—careful, fair deliberation about any conflict—is the most powerful prevention. [W. Chankim and Renée Mauborgne, Fair Process: Managing in the Knowledge Economy, *Harvard Business Review,* Jan. 2003.] Fair process keeps most people from getting a chip on their shoulder or harboring a grudge. So the easiest and most universal way to practice prevention is to use the good conflict-handling skills and techniques the wizard teaches in his guide-book and workshop.

But every now and then, the situation may get out of control. Violence does occur, and it is wise to be aware of the risk and to be sensitive to any warning signs. When someone seems out of control and primed to act violently, you should try to avoid engaging with them. If you have to, you can use your highly developed reflective listening skills and bridge to them emotionally. But that is only a good idea if you can't avoid the situation. Far better is to practice prevention by raising the alarm and making sure that care is taken to prevent them from doing any harm in the first place.

This advice is controversial. Someone may well complain that they have been "harassed" or "falsely accused" as a result of our publishing this violence prevention checklist, and of your using it. If so, sincerest apologies are more than appropriate. The problem with trying to predict workplace violence is that you inevitably will get "false positives," or indicators of trouble that turn out not to have been valid. Does this mean we should give up and not try to protect ourselves and our coworkers from possible dangers? Certainly not!

When it comes to workplace (or family) violence (or to terrorism or any other threat to the common good), it is better to be safe than sorry. Take reasonable steps to keep everyone safe and sound. That's what a conflict wizard would do. And if it is done with sensitivity and care, then should you be wrong, at least you can fall back on the fact that you used reasonable criteria and did your best for the common good. What more can we expect of any conflict wizard?

Parting Thoughts

A good rule of thumb that comes from studying incidents of workplace violence is,

Never ignore a conflict dragon.

Dragons do not go away on their own. It takes active effort—wizard skills and actions—to resolve any conflict.

This is just as true of the many productive or non-dangerous conflicts as it is of the rare conflict that can lead to violence. Conflicts should not be ignored! They are an important focus of our efforts, whether we are working on a job, a relationship, or a broader issue in the political or social sphere. The wizard has enough "conflict magic" from his or her training to be able to tackle most conflicts without anxiety, uncertainty or fear.

Things always go more smoothly when conflicts are acknowledged quickly and given sufficient attention to bring them to a reasonable and fair resolution for all concerned. Please use your skills to recognize and resolve conflicts, even if others around you seem reluctant to do so. Your good example will spread like a ripple on a pond, helping those around you to handle conflicts more productively too.

Endnotes

1 Police report statistics cited in *Training*, March 2000. Trust data from 1999 Hudson Institute Survey and from Jeffrey Pfeffer of Stanford University.

2 U.S. Center for Disease Control data, summarized in Henry Goldman, The Soaring Cost of Gun Violence, *Bloomberg*, May 2000 (see p.71). (The rates of U.S. shooting deaths and injuries are about twice those in France, four times those of Canada, and ten times those of England.)

3 You'll learn a conflict-handling approach in the coming pages that is based on communication skills. Road rage is the one area where it does not work very well, because one of the main causes of road rage incidents is that people cannot communicate as well and clearly in cars as person to person. If you want to understand other's road rage, and defuse your own, keep in mind that people cannot see or hear each other very well when in cars. Remembering that you are trying to deal with interpersonal issues "blind" when in traffic helps you maintain your patience and sense of humor about it.

4 Roy J. Lewicki, Alexander Hiam, and Karen Wise Olander, *Think Before You Speak: A Complete Guide to Strategic Negotiation*, Wiley, 1996, p.70. K. Thomas and R. Killman, *The Conflict Mode Inventory*, XICOM, 1974. (Note for 2 nd Edition: Now published by Consulting Psychologists Press.)

5 *Dealing with Conflict Instrument*, Alexander Hiam, HRD Press (Amherst MA), 1999.

6 "Collaboration is particularly appropriate in the following situations: Within an organization; When two parties have common ground; In situations where two parties have the same customers, same clients, same suppliers, or same service personnel. In any of these cases, the parties have or want to establish a working relationship and want to keep it working smoothly. In addition, we strongly recommend collaboration whenever the obvious outcomes of a negotiation are undesirable to the players. If you are all fighting over a small pie, the temptation is to compete all the harder. But...if you use collaboration to search for new and better approaches to the conflict—treating it as a puzzle rather than a fight—then you are likely to improve the outcomes for both parties." Roy J. Lewicki and Alexander Hiam, *The Fast-Forward MBA in Negotiating and Deal Making*, Wiley, 1999, pages 150-151.

7 "Participants in our courses tell us that one of the most difficult things about collaborative problem solving is the fact that they are often unaware they need this skill at the start of an interaction because they are unaware of the other person's needs." Robert Bolton, *People Skills: How to Assert Yourself, Listen to Others, and Resolve Conflicts*, Simon & Schuster, 1979, p.243. (Also, on p. 242, "Often...the conflict of needs is camouflaged. One or both parties may be unaware of the other person's need at the outset of the conversation.") Additional notes for second edition: The fact that we often are unaware of another person's needs is perhaps an artifact of our modern society, in which people have a lot more privacy and a lot less intimacy than was historically common. As Carl Rogers has observed, "We in the West seem to have made a fetish out of complete individual self-sufficiency, of not needing help, of being completely private except in a very few selected relationships. This way of living would have been completely impossible during most of history, but modern technology makes this goal achievable. With my private room, private car, private office, private (and preferably unlisted) telephone, with food and clothing purchased in large impersonal stores, with my own stove, refrigerator, dishwasher, washer-dryer, I can be practically immune from intimate contact with any other person...The utmost in privacy of personal life can be— and often is—achieved. We have reached our goal. But we pay a price." Carl R. Rogers, *A Way of Being*, Houghton Mifflin, 1980, p. 199. One price is that people do not know enough about each other to be fully aware of each others' underlying interests, and so it is perhaps more necessary now than historically to employ advanced reflective listening skills to find out what others need— or to set the stage for sharing our own essential requirements with others.

8 Peter McKellar, The Emotion of Anger in the Expression of Human Aggressiveness, *British Journal of Psychology* 39, 1949, and John Sabini, Aggression in the Laboratory, in Kutash et al. Eds., *Violence*, Jossey-Bass, 1978.

9 "Needs are open-ended, solutions are closed. Trying to impose solutions is not a way to win friends or resolve conflicts." So "...define the problem in terms of participant needs (rather than solutions)." David A Lax and James K. Sebenius, Interests: The Measure of Negotiation, *Negotiation Journal*, January 1986. Yet, we often enter a conflict assuming that the other party's positions and interests are closed-ended and directly opposed to our own (whereas they may not be that much in opposition, and may be somewhat more flexible than we assume). Two quotes from Roger Fisher et al., *Beyond Machiavelli: Tools for Coping with Conflict*, Penguin Books, 1996, illustrate these important points: "In taking positions, we tend to assume that an adversary's interests and ours are directly opposed. For instance, if we care about security, we will t̶h̶i̶s̶ ̶a̶s̶s̶u̶m̶e̶ ̶t̶h̶a̶t̶ ̶o̶t̶h̶e̶r̶s̶ ̶w̶a̶n̶t̶ ̶t̶o̶ ̶h̶a̶r̶m̶ ̶u̶s̶.̶ ̶I̶f̶ ̶w̶e̶ ̶f̶e̶e̶l̶ ̶i̶n̶s̶e̶c̶u̶r̶e̶ ̶a̶b̶o̶u̶t̶ ̶o̶u̶r̶ ̶o̶r̶i̶g̶i̶n̶s̶, we may assume that others want to push us around" (p. 36). And also, "In order to serve our own interest and to maximize the chances for a peaceful and orderly accommodation [he uses the term broadly to mean resolution], we want to preserve some flexibility in the options we propose. This flexibility will enable us to craft options that meet a broader number of our underlying interests—and theirs as well" (p. 37).

Max H. Bazeman also addresses the limitations of most people's initial views of a conflict, framing this is terms of whether they take a "fixed-pie" (distributive) or, better, an "integrative" viewpoint. Here Bazeman is quoted at length from Why Negotations Go Wrong, *Psychology Today Magazine,* 1986 (the article also is reproduced in Ira and Sandra Asherman, *The Negotiation Sourcebook*, HRD Press, 1990):

> Two sisters have a single orange to share. One wants to make orange juice. The other wants the peel to make a cake. After much discussion, they agree to a distributive compromise. They each take half the orange and end up with a very small glass of juice for one sister and a very small cake for the other.

> In this example, first presented by Mary Follett many years ago, the sisters overlooked an integrative solution: One sister takes all the juice and the other takes all the peel. This way, each gets exactly what she wants and twice as much as she received. Such integrative solutions reconcile the parties' interests and yield a higher joint benefit than is possible through simple compromise. Unfortunately, too many negotiators have the same "fixed-pie" bias that kept the sisters fighting over the orange: They assume that there is only a fixed amount of profit or gain in what is being negotiated and that in order for them to win something, the other party must necessarily lose it.

Bazeman concludes that "This is true in some negotiations, of course, but too often we assume it is without trying to think integratively." He attributes the lack of integrative thinking in our approach to the traditions of "our highly competitive society," and he cites experiences such as athletics, school admissions and job promotions as examples of competitive experiences. Thus, he argues, "Faced with negotiations that require both competition and cooperation, *as most do*, we think only of the competitive aspects. This orientation produces a distributive rather than an integrative approach to bargaining." (Emphasis added.)

10 The most successful negotiators ask at least twice as many questions in a conflict as the average person, and they are "non-linear" in their approach—they don't impose a strict sequence or process, but instead let their exploration of the underlying issues guide them. Neil Racham, The Behavior of Successful Negotiators, in Roy Lewicki et al., *Negotiation: Readings, Exercises and Cases*, 2nd Edition, Irwin, 1993. "Here's what people who are slow to anger do naturally: they empathize with the provocateur's behavior and try to find justifications for it." Carol Tavris, *Anger: The Misunderstood Emotion*, Simon & Schuster, 1982, p. 147. Also, see Robert Bolton, *People Skills: How to Assert Yourself, Listen to Others, and Resolve Conflicts*, Simon & Schuster, 1979, for detailed coverage of basic reflective listening skills. Bolton also makes the interesting observation that, "Many people find it ironic that good listening could involve interrupting the person doing the talking..." but "after a few interruptions, the speaker and I develop a rhythm of speaking and reflection that promotes better conversation" and "the speaker usually stops talking in circles and usually moves much more directly to the point." (Page. 96.) Also note the relevance of "reappraisal" strategies, which the Wizard's approach to reflective listening takes advantage of. By leading us to identify root causes of others' irritating behaviors, reflective listening helps defuse our own frustrations and puts us in a more empathetic and clear-headed frame of mind, ready for collaborative problem-solving. See Raymond W. Novaco, *Anger Control*, D.C. Heath, Lexington Books, 1975, and Ann Frodi, Effects of Varying Explanations Given for a Provocation on Subsequent Hostility, *Psychological Reports* 38, April 1976.

11 Elliot Aronson et al., *Social Psychology*, Third Edition, Addison Wesley Longman, 1999, p. 486.

12 "Defending and attacking were often difficult to distinguish from each other. What one negotiator perceived as a legitimate defense, the other party might see as an unwarranted attack. This was the root cause of most defending/attacking spirals..." Neil Rackham, The Behavior of Successful Negotiators, in Roy Lewicki et al., *Negotiation: Readings, Exercises and Cases*, 2nd Edition, Irwin, 1993. In Rackham's comparisons of exceptional and average negotiators, the exceptional ones avoided even relatively mild defensive talk such as "You can't blame us for that," or "It's not our fault." Rackham reports that "such comments frequently provoked a sharp defensive reaction from the other side of the table."

13 Leigh Thompson, Negotiation Behavior and Outcomes: Empirical Evidence and Theoretical Issues, *Psychological Bulletin* 108, 1990, and *The Mind and Heart of the Negotiator*, Prentice Hall, 1997.

14 Retaliation is not cathartic and does not reduce feelings of anger or aggressive behavior according to Carolyn Atkinson and Janet Polivy, Effects of Delay, Attack and Retaliation on State Depression and Hostility, *Journal of Abnormal Psychology* 85(6), December 1976. And Michael Kahn finds that people remain angrier with someone after expressing their anger in The Physiology of Catharsis, *Journal of Personality and Society* 3(3), 1966. Also, trying to "outdo" your opponent builds hostility on both sides, and you can't lower your opponent's hostility until you control yours first, according to Don Fitz and Maureen Findley, Anger Between Women and Men: Effects of Four Counteraggression Strategies, paper presented to American Psychological Association, 1979. And Robert Kaplan finds that expressing anger makes people more hostile than expressing neutral or concerned attitudes in The Cathartic Value of Self-Expression: Testing Catharsis, Dissonance, and Interference Explanations, *Journal of Social Psychology* 97(2), December 1975.]

Additional notes for the second edition: Also, in a general sense, being calm rather than angry is "good for business" because people do not like to deal with other people who are not in control of their emotions. Daniel Goleman summarizes the research on this important point in *Working with Emotional Intelligence*, Bantam Books, 1998, p. 176: "Being in control of our own moods is also essential to good communication. A study of 130 executives and managers found that how well people handled their own emotions determined the degree to which those around them preferred to deal with them. In dealing with peers and subordinates, calmness and patience were key. Bosses likewise preferred dealing with employees who were not overly aggressive with them...Aiming for a neutral mood is the best strategy in anticipation of dealing with someone else, if only because it makes us an emotional clean slate and allows us to adapt to whatever the situation calls for."

The idea that catharsis, or "venting," is an effective response to conflicts, or to anger in general, is ingrained in our culture and many others. It is important to make clear that this is a myth. Yes, even in this modern, scientific society, we still do have myths. For instance, the vast majority of people believe that among 'primitive' groups, cannibalism was common. This is a myth, not a fact, as the anthropologist W. A. Arens has shown in *The Man-eating Myth: Anthropology and Anthropophagy,* Oxford University Press, 1979, and yet most people will argue vehemently that cannibalism is true and not mythological. People also believe firmly that venting, or expressing your anger, is a helpful thing to do, in spite of decades of studies showing that it is a serious mistake. Goleman has reviewed the evidence against catharsis, tracing back more than thirty years, yet the popular viewpoint still holds that venting is a good idea. Here is what Goleman found, as quoted from *Emotional Intelligence*, Bantam Books, 1995, p. 64: "Catharsis—giving vent to rage—is sometimes extolled as a way of handling anger. The popular theory holds that "it makes you feel better." But, as Zillerman's findings suggest, there is an argument against catharsis. It has been made since the 1950s, when psychologists started to test the effects of catharsis experimentally and, time after time, found that giving vent to anger did little or nothing to dispel it (although, because of the seductive nature of anger, it may *feel* satisfying)." [Goleman cites Mallick and McCandless, A Study of Catharsis Aggression, in *Journal of Personality and Social Psychology* 4 (1996).] Also, Goleman points out in his review (pp. 64-65) that, "Tice found that ventilating anger is one of the worst ways to cool down: outbursts of rage typically pump up the emotional brain's arousal, leaving people feeling more angry, not less." Yet, as Goleman points out, anger can be "seductive," or perhaps more accurately (for the effect is on ourselves and not others), addictive. It is important to admit that the myth of catharsis is just that, a myth, and that to truly manage conflicts well, we must give up on our addictive attraction to the notion that it is okay to vent our anger. If you cannot stop venting, then make sure you do it in private and "get it out of your system" fully *before* you interact with others. And even then, you must guard against the contaminating effects of venting, for it is likely to bias you negatively toward the imagined source or cause of you anger.

15 "Our experience of assertion training with thousands of people leads us to conclude that repeated small irritants often grow until they loom large in the feeling world. When people do not get their needs met in the commonplace trivialities of life, they build up reservoirs of resentment that diminish their acceptance of the other person...and make it far more difficult to solve the 'big' problems when they arise." Robert Bolton, *People Skills: How to Assert Yourself, Listen to Others, and Resolve Conflicts,* Simon & Schuster, 1979, p. 149.

16 Neil Rackham, The Behavior of Successful Negotiators, in Roy Lewicki et al., *Negotiation: Readings, Exercises and Cases*, 2nd Edition, Irwin, 1993.

17 Roger Fisher and Wayne H. Davis, Six Basic Interpersonal Skills for a Negotiator's Repertoire, *Negotiation Journal*, April 1987, pages 117-122. (Note: Most people are too tough on the other person in a conflict, and too soft on the underlying interests. They wear out relationships without solving problems or achieving goals.)

Index

HD 42
, H 53
2003